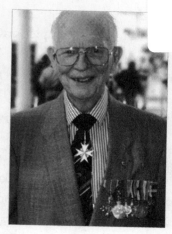

Dr Rowley Richards, MBE, OAM, ED, graduated from the University of Sydney in Medicine with MB BS in 1939, aged 23, and led a distinguished career in both medicine and the military. Following his return home to Sydney after three and a half years as a Japanese prisoner of war, Dr Richards was Mentioned in Dispatches (MID) in 1947 for his service as a regimental medical officer while imprisoned in Changi, along the Burma–Siam Railway and in Japan, and in 1969 was awarded an MBE for service in war and peace. He also earned the Efficiency Decoration (ED). He is a Foundation Fellow of the Australian College of Occupational Medicine and the Australian Sports Medicine Federation, and has also been granted fellowships by the Royal Australian College of General Practitioners, the American College of Sports Medicine and the Australian Institute of Management.

In 1960 Dr Richards joined the St John Ambulance Association, where he was heavily involved in standardising first-aid training programs for St John Ambulance examinations, and ultimately designed the St John first-aid kits based on the Army first-aid kits he had issued to his own men before going into action in the Malayan campaign. He became NSW chairman and vice president, and in 1981 was awarded a Knight of the Order of St John.

Passionate about health and fitness, after being selected as medical advisor for the Australian Olympic Rowing teams for the Mexico Games in 1968 and Munich in 1972, Dr Richards went on to hold the position of honorary medical director of the Sydney City to Surf Fun Run between 1977 and 1998. He stepped down from this role after 21 years of service and remains honorary medical consultant. In 1993 he was awarded an OAM for his service to sports medicine and the City to Surf, and in 2003 he was awarded the Australian Centenary Medal for service to the sick and injured through the St John Ambulance Association.

Dr Richards retired from his medical practice in executive health in 2000, aged 83, and now lives in Beacon Hill, Sydney, with Beth, his wife of 58 years. As president of the 2/15th Field Regiment Association and president of the 8th Australian Division Association, Dr Richards remains active and committed to caring for fellow veterans and their families, and to preserving veteran memory.

A DOCTOR'S WAR

ROWLEY RICHARDS

HarperCollins*Publishers*

HarperCollins_Publishers_

First published in Australia in 2005
by HarperCollins_Publishers_ Pty Limited
ABN 36 009 913 517
A member of the HarperCollins_Publishers_ (Australia) Pty Limited Group
www.harpercollins.com.au

HarperCollins_Publishers_
25 Ryde Road, Pymble, Sydney, NSW 2073, Australia
31 View Road, Glenfield, Auckland 10, New Zealand
77–85 Fulham Palace Road, London W6 8JB, United Kingdom
2 Bloor Street East, 20th Floor, Toronto, Ontario M4W 1A8, Canada
10 East 53rd Street, New York, NY 10022, USA

National Library of Australia Cataloguing-in-Publication data:

Richards, Rowley.
  A doctor's war.
  Bibliography.
  Includes index.
  ISBN 0 7322 8008 7.
  1. Richards, Rowley. 2. Physicians – Australia – Biography.
  3. World War, 1939–1945 – Prisoners and prisons, Japanese.
  4. World War, 1939–1945 – Personal narratives, Australian.
  5. Prisoners of war – Australia. 6. Prisoners of war – Japan.
  I. Title.
940.547252.

Cover picture: A stretch of the Burma–Siam Railway, Tampi, Thailand (Australian War Memorial
PO1910.022); and Rowley Richards
Unless otherwise noted, all pictures from Rowley Richards' private collection. Every effort has
been made to contact copyright holders and the publishers
welcome inquiries where copyright may have been infringed.
Cover and internal design by Natalie Winter, HarperCollins Design Studio
Maps by Laurie Whiddon, Map Illustrations.
Typeset in 12.5 on 16pt Bembo by Kirby Jones
Printed and bound in Australia by Griffin Press on 79gsm Bulky White

6 5 4 3   05 06 07 08

For Beth, my wife and best friend.
And for my medical orderlies,
their patients and relatives.

CONTENTS

ACKNOWLEDGMENTS

My continuing thanks go to those who provided assistance and material which has been used in the writing of this book. I particularly thank Roy Whitecross and the late John Williams who loaned me their diaries, and the relatives of the late Jim Lynch, Scippy Maher, Bill McGee and Kitch Loughnan whose diaries were made available to me.

I also thank Dr Peter Stanley, principal historian at the Australian War Memorial, Canberra, for his encouragement and for his introduction to a publisher. Shona Martyn and Helen Littleton at HarperCollins won me over with their enthusiasm, expertise and experience. They suggested that Alison Orman, a part-time senior editor with them, might be able to assist with the writing.

It has been my extreme good fortune that she accepted the proposal. With her dedication and exceptional investigative ability, this book took on a new life. She has become much more than an editor. She and her husband, Jan, have become friends — almost part of the family. Advancing pregnancy did nothing to dampen her ardour and enthusiasm for the project. As a result of her persistent questions, which made me research my diaries and documents more carefully, I became aware of many things that I had forgotten or did not fully appreciate when I wrote them down.

Bruce Kennedy as agent has helped me negotiate the path into publishing with patience and understanding. Mary Rennie, editor, and Amruta Slee, publisher, have been most helpful in their guidance of the manuscript through the maze of external editing, proofreading, printing and production as a book.

I am grateful to Andrew Denton and Dr Peter Stanley for their generous comments in the Foreword and Introduction respectively. I also thank Major General S.N. Gower, AO, Director of the Australian War Memorial (AWM), and Anne Bennie; and Ian Smith and Jennifer Coombes, from the AWM Research Department, for their cooperation and assistance with the reproduction of pictures from the Rowley Richards Collection held by the AWM. I particularly thank Jennifer for the meticulous preparation of the collection catalogue.

I especially thank Pinkey Rhodes, my last remaining medical orderly, for agreeing to be interviewed by Alison Orman, for his selfless service during action and as a prisoner of war, and most of all for his loyalty and friendship.

I am greatly in debt to the following for returning valuable items to me after the war: the late John Shaw for carrying my original diary (Part 2) in the false bottom of a billycan; to the late Jim Armstrong for maintaining my medical records and microscope; and to the Directorate of War Grave Services for sending a special squad to Pulau Damarlaut, off Singapore Island, to recover my buried diary summary and medical records. These diaries and records made it possible for me to ultimately write this book. I also thank Mary Best and the many people who have assisted with typing and expanding my diaries into a narrative form.

Above all, I thank my wife, Beth, for her participation in most of my major postwar activities and for her constant inspiration, encouragement and editorial skills at every step (or word) along the way. Our sons, David and Ian, have also maintained their support and given helpful advice. My sincere thanks to all of you.

FOREWORD

Rowley Richards does not sit comfortably in today's world of the metrosexual male, where no thought is left unexpressed, no emotional depth unplumbed.

Here is a man, by his own admission, more at home with facts than feelings. He comes from that post-Victorian era when any slip of the mask revealing what lay beneath was considered a sign of weakness.

And Rowley is a doctor: a man used to keeping meticulous and dispassionate records — symptoms, procedures, doses, results — anything but emotions.

For almost 60 years, Rowley has tried to keep things this way. To clamp a lid on the vast pit of horrors and heroics he witnessed while a Japanese POW. To never let anyone in because how could anyone possibly understand?

He even tried it in this book (it became a running joke between him and his editor: 'Yes, Rowley, but how did you feel?'). But, in spite of himself, beneath all that carefully applied veneer of detail and reserve, Rowley has written a memoir of such deep emotional strength your breath will literally be taken away.

It says something about Rowley Richards' war that contracting smallpox was one of his better moments. Here is a man, a 'cocky little bugger', captured at the fall of Singapore, aged just 26, and forced to endure deprivation and ruination to make Dante hang his head.

Down through the various circles of hell he descends, through a world where men are so frightened they try to claw through bitumen roads with their bare hands; through the death camps of the Burma Railway, with disease and humiliation as his constant companions; through a Godless world, where the pages of the Bible are only good for rolling cigarettes; and deeper still, through a world where human life, worth less than nothing, can be snuffed out on a whim, with no opportunity for justice or retaliation; down through the holds of Japanese hell ships and the torpedos that leave him adrift; through the unspeakable bitterness of a Tokyo winter, where people line the streets to laugh at his wretchedness; down, down he falls into the darkest part of the deepest pit of human cruelty.

All this is in here and the inhumanity will leave you aghast. But it is the humanity in this memoir that will make you want to weep.

In writing *A Doctor's War*, Rowley talks of fulfilling a sense of duty in honour of his comrades. He can consider the mission accomplished. While he does not shrink from recording bad, sometimes cowardly, behaviour of Allied POW's, these are very few and all the more shocking for that.

Instead, it is his portraits of men enduring barbarism with unshakable integrity that stay with you. Furtive kindnesses, subtle moments of tenderness, brief gestures of defiance — these are the small moments that dwarf the bigger picture of war's madness.

Rowley Richards and the men with whom he served would not thank you for calling them heroes. They don't see themselves that way (for many, guilt about the capitulation at Singapore never entirely went away). All they did was survive the war, not win it. In a strict military sense, that may be so, but they are heroes, nonetheless, and in a way so profound the medal has not yet been struck that can honour them.

Albert Schweitzer, who, like Rowley, understood intimately the weight of a man's soul, once observed, '*The tragedy of a man is what dies inside himself while he still lives.*' The miracle captured here is what lived inside these men while so many died.

Andrew Denton, May 2005

INTRODUCTION

One of the great pleasures of the job I am privileged to do is that it lets me meet people whose experiences I and the great majority of Australians will — thankfully — never share. Many of these people have known the trauma of war, something which most of us can only understand by entering into the memories of those able to reach us through their words. Among the hundreds of veterans I have met, Dr Rowley Richards stands out as the most impressive man.

I agreed to write this introduction under a mild protest. I felt that Rowley Richards' qualities are so much to be cherished by the people of this nation that he ought to have been introduced by someone of greater standing. Rowley has a persuasive way, though; and here I am writing it. My only excuse for accepting this task is that having met him, and having over twenty years or so learned something of his story, I can make an introduction that is based on knowledge and respect rather than out of simple courtesy or from a hastily absorbed briefing.

Rowley's story begins long before the Second World War, with a deft sketch of the family and the society in which he grew up. He evokes a long-gone Australia, one whose values he retains: indeed, values which sustained him through the ordeal he chronicles.

The story Rowley tells may sound familiar. Books by and about prisoners of the Japanese have related it before. Rowley describes the brief but costly fighting for Malaya and Singapore, the disorientation and humiliation of Changi, the unremitting labour of the Burma–Thailand Railway, and the agony of the sinking of the *Rakuyo Maru*. But however familiar these episodes may seem, we can understand them more deeply through reading *A Doctor's War*.

Rowley's recollection of these experiences tells us much that we could learn in no other way. Even if he is right, that we cannot really know unless we have supped from the same cup, we can glimpse something of what it must have been like to choose sick men to work on the Railway, for example, or lie exhausted upon the deck of a Japanese ship, not knowing whether it would be torpedoed. The restrained, reflective tone in which he tells his story adds immeasurably to its authenticity and power.

A Doctor's War is only the latest of Rowley's services. He worked as a doctor in war and captivity and as a civilian medical practitioner for over 50 years. He has served his fellow former prisoners of war as president of the cohesive and energetic 2/15th Field Regiment Association for nearly 60 years. He has carefully collated his papers, now held in the Research Centre of the Australian War Memorial, which allow us to understand more deeply his story and our history.

Finally, he has now taken the trouble to write a powerful and moving record of his wartime experience. *A Doctor's War* reminds us of what he and his fellow prisoners faced — one of the greatest challenges which have ever confronted a group of Australians — and how he and they met it: with good-humour, compassion and courage.

A Doctor's War is not only valuable as an historical record. It is also — perhaps above all — a moving document of humanity. Rowley Richards' own qualities shine through his story: candour, humility, a capacity for self-deprecating humour and a deep insight into and sympathy for the human condition. He tells a story which deserves to endure.

Peter Stanley
Principal Historian
Australian War Memorial

IN 2001, DR ROWLEY RICHARDS *donated his personal papers to the Australian War Memorial (including parts of his original wartime diaries and buried diary summary and medical records), known as the Rowley Richards Collection (AWM PR01916). For further information, including a guide to the collection, visit www.awm.gov.au.*

PROLOGUE

I remember clearly the day my long-lost diary summary was returned to me. It was 15 February 1947, the fifth anniversary of the fall of Singapore. The events of the disastrous Malayan campaign and our surrender had been playing through my mind all day, like fragments of a film: from the long march to Birdwood Camp in Changi to the horrors that followed throughout my three and a half years as a Japanese prisoner of war. I had been back home in Australia for almost sixteen months by then and was enjoying living my life to the full, making up for lost time. I was 31 years old and working as a resident doctor at Crown Street Women's Hospital in Sydney.

That evening, still wearing my white coat, stethoscope dangling from my neck, I walked into my residents' quarters within the hospital. Exhausted after finishing another long shift on the wards, I was looking forward to supper, a nip of scotch and then sleep. As I entered the sitting room, I noticed a large, official-looking brown envelope propped up against the wall behind the mantelpiece, where our housekeeper always left mail for the doctors. Curious, I straightened my spectacles and walked over to look at it. Addressed to me in neatly typed letters, it was stamped with 'On Her Majesty's Service' and the sender was 'The Directorate of War Graves Services'.

With an expectation of pleasure (in fact, I don't think I have ever looked forward more to anything in my life), I opened the envelope without delay. Inside was a letter clipped to a thin bundle of loose pages. It read:

> *Dear Doctor,*
>
> *With reference to your letter of 25th June 1946, and your more recent visit to this office, I am now pleased to enclose the notes which you buried under Cpl. Gorlick's grave cross.*
>
> *I hope you find them intact and are able to make good use of them.*
>
> *Yours faithfully,*
> *D. A. Wright Sq. / Ldr.*
> *Directorate of War Graves Services*

I counted the attached pages: seven sheets in total plus a larger sheet summarising my medical records, as well as an old Red Cross envelope. It was all there; my buried treasure had at last been uncovered.

I had been waiting for this moment since 11 August 1944, the day I had buried a detailed summary of my war diaries beneath a wooden cross that marked the grave of Corporal Gorlick, one of our many men who died during captivity. At that time, I had been a prisoner of war for two and a half years; we had endured cruelty, starvation, disease, impossible working conditions, violence and murder. The Burma–Siam Railway had been completed and my prisoner group (Kumi No. 35 — we were always known by numbers, never a name) was en route from the island of Singapore to labour camps in Japan. I knew my journey ahead involved a perilous voyage across the torpedo-infested South China Sea. I had not lost hope of surviving but by that point I had accepted death might well be imminent. Convinced there was a high probability my contraband diaries would soon end up in Japanese hands — lost forever — I had made the decision to bury a detailed summary of my writings and records.

I could hardly believe I was now holding these same pages in my hands. Apart from a slight yellowing of the paper, they were in remarkably fine condition. After telephoning friends and family to tell them the good news, I retired to my bedroom where I hoped to remain uninterrupted for the rest of the evening. I cracked open a bottle of scotch, filled my pipe with Ranch tobacco and sat up in my single bed, a pillow behind my back, ready to savour my own history. I began to read every word, left to right, line by line, something I have done repeatedly over the years since.

I cannot tell you, in specific terms, the feelings I experienced when I was reunited with my buried pages. I was excited, of course, I'm sure my hands must have been trembling as I read, but that you would expect. I am much more comfortable with facts than feelings. I find it easier to recall the precise dimensions of a house I once lived in rather than tell you what it felt like to live inside. I am a stickler for the truth; a list keeper; and at times a pedant. I do not like revealing or losing control of my emotions: it is a practice of self-preservation I was forced to perfect as a prisoner of war, and it has remained with me ever since.

I am now 89 years old and still each time I read my pages I cannot remember all of the events my words allude to. I find my own experiences highly unlikely, yet I have proof in the blue ink of my summary notes; facts I can grip on to and trust far more than my own memories. When re-reading my writings, I often feel detached, as if I am following someone else's journey through war and captivity. Sometimes I even find myself thinking, 'those poor buggers were really having a terrible time', without seeing myself as one of them. For most of my life I have successfully distanced myself from some of my worst experiences, blunting the emotions.

My lack of recall has, at times, confounded me. Of course there are possible medical explanations — cerebral damage from malnutrition or repeated and prolonged exposure to psychic trauma — but I have always suspected that many of my memories were not permanently lost but rather locked away for safe keeping. I survived the Burma–Siam Railway and a shipwreck in the South China Sea, yet following the end of the war, the memories I recalled were largely based on humorous incidents, events involving my mates; stories which demonstrated brotherly love, compassion, self-sacrifice and devotion to one's fellow man. Recollections of mateship in its truest sense. Meanwhile, neatly packaged and shelved in another part of my mind, were private and protected thoughts of the misery, brutality and degradation of life in captivity. I learned to block out certain events in order to survive, to move on and lead a meaningful life free of bitterness or regret — two particular states of mind I believe will only ever lead a person nowhere fast. It is only in recent years that I have slowly allowed emotions to surface. I can now shed tears and acknowledge some of my darker moments in ways I couldn't as a younger man who still had the rest of his life ahead of him. Little by little, my barriers have dropped — at least somewhat.

In the following pages, I tell my story based upon the facts recorded in my diaries and medical records, and the memories my mind allows me to call upon. The most enduring responsibility for those of us who survived at the hands of the Imperial Japanese Army is to do all in our power to ensure that our experiences are not forgotten and never repeated. Every prisoner of war has his own story to tell; I can only offer you mine. My story is not one that should evoke pity; it is a story of survival through senseless suffering and, above all else, of hope and optimism. I trust it will also serve as a form of remembrance to the valour and dignity of my comrades and mates, especially my medical orderlies.

PART ONE

BEGINNINGS

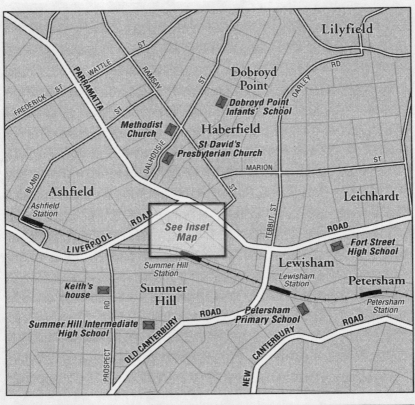

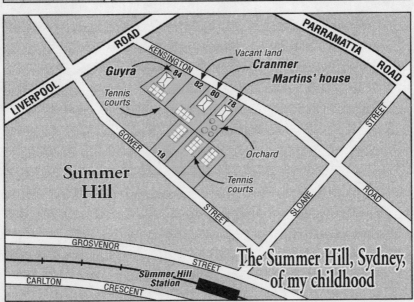

The Summer Hill, Sydney, of my childhood

CHAPTER ONE

A QUIET BOYHOOD

My very first memory of childhood is not pleasant. I was about three years old when Dr Campbell, a friendly, rotund Scotsman, arrived on the doorstep of our family home in Sydney's Summer Hill, his well-worn black medical bag in hand. After brief welcoming pleasantries between the good doctor and my parents it was time to get down to business in our lounge room. Dr Campbell bent down and lifted me up onto the edge of my father's billiard table. 'There we go, boy. Be with you in a tick.'

I sat upright, my chubby legs dangling over the side of the table. I watched this jolly man setting out his metal kidney dishes and shiny instruments in a neat row beside me, my blue eyes alight with wonder. I had no idea he intended to use his tools on me. My mother, always prepared, had covered the billiard table with a large cloth to avoid potential mess. I can still remember Dr Campbell gently placing an ether mask over my face before I drifted off into darkness, his kindly voice assuring me: 'You won't feel a thing.'

When I awoke sometime later, flat on my back on the billiard table, blinking at the ceiling, I had an awful burning sensation in my groin. I sat up and looked downwards to find my penis wrapped up like a sore thumb. The pain lasted for weeks; I'll never forget it — physical pain can often be easier to recall than other forms of suffering. Circumcision was my rude initiation into the world of medicine.

MY PARENTS ALWAYS HOPED I would one day become a doctor. The first words my father uttered when my arrival was announced to him on 8 June 1916 were: 'And he shall be a doctor.' He sometimes repeated these words to me during my childhood, but he didn't hammer them in as an ultimatum. My mother, suitably proud that several of her ancestors had been surgeons in the Royal Navy, also believed medicine would be an appropriate career choice for me; but, like my father, her wishes were implicit rather than overt.

That my parents ever spoke a word at all was astonishing. Both were completely deaf, and yet they could speak clearly. They also were able to lip-read. My father, Charles Howell Richards, was born deaf as a result of his mother developing rubella during pregnancy. My mother, curiously named Clive Bromley, became deaf at about age three due to complications of diphtheria. My mother was teaching deaf children to speak at the Deaf and Dumb School in Sydney when she met my father, who was then a lay preacher at the Adult Deaf and Dumb Society. They married in 1915.

My father worked as a draughtsman for Sydney's leading cartographer, H.E.C. Robinson, who drew much of the original Sydney street directory today known as *Gregory's*. Despite the Depression, he was never out of work. H.E.C. Robinson ensured each of his employees had at least one day's work a week; none of his men went without a pay packet. My father's deafness enabled him to do his exacting job with maximum concentration. Sometimes when he was working from home I would sit beside him and watch. Using a pencil, he drafted topographical features and printing marks onto large sheets of transparent linen before drawing his final maps freehand, aided by a roller ruler, in permanent black ink. He could labour away for hours on end and achieve absolute accuracy. I learned by example that there was only one way to carry out your work — meticulously.

My mother was terribly proper. She was forever telling me, 'Rowley, it's not *proper* to do such and such.' Her favourite maxim was: 'Trust in God and fear no man.' She never left the house without her hat, a hat pin neatly fixed to one side. A very contained person, she didn't rely on anyone but herself. She had a sweet, smiling face — the proper face a woman was expected to have on public display in those days — which shielded a sometimes wicked temper. Despite her ardent sense of respectability, she still knew how to have fun, and how to make the most of her disability. I remember when we visited the local butcher's shop, we would stand outside the front window, me holding her hand by her side, until the butcher noticed us. When he did, he grinned before raising one hand to his shoulder — *tap* — 'Do you want a shoulder of lamb today, Mrs Richards?' My mother would nod or shake her head. Then he would move his hand to his thigh — *tap, tap* — 'How about a leg roast?' And then his backside — *tap, tap, tap* — 'Do you want some rump?'

We lived in a modest brick house with a slate-tiled roof at 80 Kensington Road, Summer Hill, throughout all of my childhood. Grandmother Polson, my father's mother, lived right next door with her second husband, Alfred Polson, a shop assistant, and their daughter, Linda. (My grandmother's first husband, Charles Howell Richards Senior, had passed away in 1887 when she was just three months pregnant with my father.) Like my mother, Grandmother Polson had very definite ideas about what was proper. She wore long black frocks that buttoned up to her neck and reached right to the ground; I never saw her legs. When my father announced he was engaged to my mother, Grandmother set about subdividing her own block of land and having a house built for my parents to live in after they were married. She named our house Cranmer, probably after the first Protestant Archbishop of Canterbury. It had two bedrooms, a bathroom, a kitchen-laundry where my mother kept her copper, and a drawing room, which became my bedroom when my brother Frank arrived four years after me. Taking pride of place in our lounge room was the billiard-cum-operating table, complete with large wooden covers. It was here that my father spread out his large rolls of transparent linen when he was working from home. Back then, it was considered necessary for a gentleman to have a billiard table, so Grandmother Polson bought one for my father (well before the Depression set in).

Grandmother Polson was a constant in my life. She exerted her loving authority from the moment I was born. When my parents christened me Rowland Bromley Richards, she protested vehemently, insisting that 'Charles', my father and grandfather's name, be formally added to the mix. Since she lived right next door, there was no escaping her disapproval, so my parents, eager for peace, quickly relented. They returned to the local minister's office and I was officially re-named 'Charles Rowland Bromley Richards'. But it didn't make any difference: I became known to all and sundry as 'Rowley' — as in the well-loved Beatrix Potter tale *The Roly-poly Pudding* — due to my tubby appearance.

WHEN I STARTED SCHOOL at Dobroyd Point Infants', two kilometres away from home, I had to learn to navigate my way across busy Liverpool and Parramatta Roads, and then down a long street to the Haberfield shopping centre, where there was a tramline. I had to cross the tramline and walk another half kilometre to school. Aunt Linda, who still lived next door with Grandmother Polson, showed me the way the first few times. After that, I was on my own. I was only four years old. It was not a case of neglect; my parents simply encouraged me to be uncommonly independent at a very early age. My mother had lost both of her parents as a young girl and my father's father had died before he was even born. There is an old saying that you learn how to be parents from your parents; my parents didn't have that luxury. In their world, children needed to be self-sufficient to survive. I remember seeing other mums, aunties and grandmothers taking their kids to school day in and day out, hands held tightly, and I used to think they were sissies. My parents led by example that you didn't need to depend on others for help. They taught me that I could achieve anything in life I wanted to, as long as I set my mind to it. It was just a matter of setting my goals and applying myself. I think this was one of the most valuable lessons I learned from them, and the fact that they were both handicapped and were still able to achieve was always an inspiration to me.

At home, my parents used sign language to communicate with each other, so I picked it up very quickly. They spoke out loud to my brother, Frank, and me and we usually mouthed our words in reply so they could lip-read; if there was any confusion we used sign language as our fallback. We also developed our own family language of shorthand signs: for example, we touched our chest in a certain way to indicate we were tired, or our forehead to let them know we had a headache. Both my parents were obsessive about perfecting their speech. Whenever they came across a new word they would practise it at home, repeating the word out loud to Frank and me until we told them they had it just right. Their voices were a little lower than normal and a touch monotone but their speech was so good they could carry on conversations in shops without shop assistants realising they were deaf. My father carried a little pocket notebook and pencil wherever he went. Because his job required absolute precision he didn't hesitate to confirm details in writing, just to make sure, but my mother did not feel the need to do the same. Sometimes my father took me

7

to work functions or meetings when he anticipated lip-reading from the audience might be impossible. I sat beside him and translated, via mouthing and sign language. If there was ever a problem for my father in communicating, he always found a solution, usually in the form of me or his notepad. His disability never stopped him from doing what he wanted.

Outside of school, weekends were consistently filled with tennis. At the rear of our narrow backyard, beyond the outside dunny, lay a loam tennis court. Nearly everyone in the neighbourhood had one — it was not a sign of wealth but more an indication that land in Sydney was not yet at a premium. One of my weekly chores was to water the court and then compact the loam with a big heavy roller. My father and I would do this together on Saturday mornings and then mark the lines; we had a machine that we used to push, its little wheels spinning out white lime as we moved along.

Every Saturday my parents hosted a tennis competition at our house for members of the Adult Deaf and Dumb Society. Saturday morning we prepared the courts; Saturday afternoon I played in district competition. My parents preferred the company of the deaf community to other families in the area. Their disability was referred to as 'deaf and dumb' because many ignorant people assumed that dumb meant stupid rather than mute. I remember watching people in the neighbourhood hesitating to start a conversation with my mother or father, unsure of whether they should speak very loudly or very slowly; most were so self-conscious about doing the wrong thing that they just didn't bother communicating with us at all. Because of this I didn't ask friends to come home to play; I was worried that they, too, would feel awkward around my parents, I wasn't embarrassed because of my parents, I just wasn't equipped yet to deal with other people's discomfort about their disability.

Despite not inviting friends over to my own home, I did spend a lot of time at the house of our neighbours, Clem and Ivy

Martin. Ivy had two sisters who both sang very well; they used to gather around the piano and have some great parties. I was frequently a welcome guest, handing around the grog for them. My visits became a scheduled daily ritual. My mother put our family meal on the table at six o'clock every night — and if you weren't there, bad luck — then, at half past six, I dashed next door to the Martins' and stayed to chat with them until seven o'clock, when it was homework time. Conversation in my own home was limited, always 'proper', I suppose. The Martins, especially Ivy, had a keen sense of humour and the banter seemed endless — something which, because of my parents' disability, was absent from my own home. With no children of their own, I think I filled a void in the lives of the Martins, just as they did in mine. They were like second parents to me, and their home was one of the few in the neighbourhood I visited.

I have often been asked if I felt different because my parents were deaf. At the time, it was the only family life I knew, and it was a happy one, but I was aware that our family was not like others. When friends introduced me to a new kid in the neighbourhood they would start with 'This is Rowley', and often follow up with 'his parents are deaf and dumb', as if it were essential information. I learned to be content in my own company. I wasn't a recluse — I enjoyed playing tennis with the other kids in our neighbourhood — but I was more than happy to come home and play on my own. I don't recall feeling lonely or ostracised; spending time on my own simply became a habit I started to enjoy. What saddened me was watching others underestimate my parents. It marked the beginning of my understanding of prejudice, even if I didn't know the right word for it as a child.

Being different also equated in some people's view to our family as underprivileged, even though compared to a lot of others during the Depression we were quite fortunate: we always had food on the table. This way of thinking was also true of most of our relatives. Aunt Leila, my mother's sister, was married to Uncle Frank, a big-time Charlie in the wool industry, and every time we visited them Uncle Frank would discreetly press two bob inside my hand as I was walking out the door. They were kind to us and very well meaning but it was obvious to me, even from a very young age, that we were seen as the poor relations. This only made me even more resolute to work hard, to show them all that I was as good as, or better than, them. It sparked in me a stubborn determination to rise above what others saw as obstacles — a trait I would understand more fully in years to come.

IN 1924 I TURNED eight and was given my first (and only) childhood birthday party. By this time, Grandmother and Grandfather Polson and Aunt Linda had moved house, but they were still within cooee distance at 19 Gower Street. Their new house, Lochnagar, stood back-to-back with Cranmer. It was also the year my father left for a six-month overseas adventure — a very unusual event at the time, and one of the most significant of my childhood. Some of my father's relations from Nottingham in England had raised money to purchase him a round-the-world ticket and my mother encouraged him to take advantage of such an extraordinary opportunity. My father was a great letter writer and had always stayed in touch with relations in England; they held a special affection and sympathy for him because he had never known his own father and because he was deaf. Back then, people rarely travelled, even among the better heeled in our neighbourhood. I knew of no one who had been abroad. For my father to be setting off overseas was a very big deal, and one that no one in our family begrudged him. So off he sailed on a passenger liner, to see the world. I still have a copy of his diary. He kept a meticulous record of his voyage, recording the ship's latitude and longitude daily, as well as precisely how far the ship had travelled in the previous 24 hours. He travelled to Colombo, Suez, watched Mt Etna erupt, visited family in the UK and then travelled across Canada on the Canadian–Pacific Railway.

My father had no problems communicating with others throughout his travels. He was a thorough gentleman, a product of the mid-Victorian era, but he was not a shy man. He would wear fancy dress at any party opportunity and he was a master at card tricks; he knew how to entertain an audience. We received vivid accounts of his journey through his letters and I knew he was coming home so was not overly concerned by his absence. I shared the joy of his travels through his writings: he opened up a whole new world of possibilities for me and filled me with a spirit of adventure that would stay with me for the rest of my life.

When he returned six months later, life in Summer Hill went on much the same as it always had. I spent most of my free time playing tennis or next door visiting the Martins. I continued to follow Grandmother and Grandfather Polson to St David's Presbyterian Church in nearby Haberfield every Sunday, just I had been doing since I was a young schoolboy. Where we lived, you were either a Catholic or a Protestant, which reflected the predominantly Anglo-Saxon population in Sydney at the time. There was a very strong anti-Catholic bias among Protestant families, and vice versa. Protestants marrying Catholics was taboo; if a couple of mixed faith insisted on marrying, one had to convert to the other's religion. In hushed voices locals would then spread the news that someone 'had turned'.

Grandfather Polson, a rabid Presbyterian, made us cross the road at a brisk pace if he saw a Catholic walking towards us on the same side. I remember one particular Sunday the Presbyterian minister at St David's said something during a service to which Grandfather took great offence. I was too young to comprehend what it was that upset him so greatly, but I remember him grabbing Grandmother's hand, who in turn snatched mine, and we got up and left mid-service. During our stride home we passed a Baptist Church, and Grandfather took us inside. He didn't much like it, so on we walked until we found a Methodist Church; in we went and in we stayed. From that point to my university days I attended Methodist Sunday School, but I only turned up because I had to. I enjoyed the companionship and recognised it as a legitimate excuse to meet girls, but I was never a believer.

The experiences with Grandfather set me firmly against bigotry, and I vowed that when I was older I would make it my business to meet as many Catholics as I could. My visits to the Martins' next door also greatly influenced my opinion of religion. They were not churchgoers, yet to me they were a loving couple who led meaningful lives and were never harsh in their judgments of others. As a young boy, I liked their way of life much better than that of Grandfather Polson. To me, faith in oneself was the most important belief you could have. At a very young age I became determined to live a good rather than religious life. Religion was just another form of prejudice; no different from the way so many in the hearing world discriminated against my parents. Of course, I kept my views to myself. Back then a boy did not argue with his elders. To speak out against religion would have been unforgivable; instead, I learned the value of silence, of restraining unspoken words at the back of my throat and hiding my opinion to avoid reproach.

I FOUND A BEST friend, Keith Elphinstone, when I started at Summer Hill Intermediate High School: Keith and I were equally mad about maths and chemistry. He was quite a serious-looking kid with brown hair that was always neatly parted to one side. We played tennis together on Saturdays and then I used to go to his house for tea most Saturday nights. Mr Elphinstone was a senior executive at a timber company so they were quite well off. Mrs Elphinstone had a Fiat Tourer, a seven-seater, and every week she used to drive this big old thing miles to a butcher's shop in Abbotsford to buy the most delicious sausages. She would arrive home with a white-paper parcel tucked under her arm and disappear into the kitchen to cook up a big plate of sausages with a tomato and onion mix. Keith had a sister and a brother, so their house was always filled with their friends eagerly awaiting her weekly treat. Visiting Keith's house made me aware of the difference between other households and ours. Keith's place was always busy — and very, very noisy.

Keith shared my passion for all things to do with aviation and technology. At the age of about ten, I entered a competition run by a Sydney newspaper. The editor printed an aerial picture of an undisclosed location in Sydney, and to win you had to identify where the photo was taken and then fill in the appropriate street names. The prize was a joy flight over Sydney in a Tiger Moth. I had an unfair advantage with my father's cartography skills available on tap, and I didn't hesitate to exploit it. (One of my early schoolteachers used to say to us: 'It's not a matter of never doing anything wrong; it's a matter of never getting caught.' Which was advice I have always been happy to follow.) My father helped me identify the area in the photograph and then dutifully brought home the relevant street map from his office. I filled in the street names and won. Such a small victory — and assisted! — but it remains one of my fondest memories of childhood. Without hesitation, I called up the editor of the newspaper to claim my prize and said: 'I'm only small, do you think I could please bring my friend along?' I reasoned that two halves make a whole. To my absolute delight, he agreed. So I took Keith, who was equally ecstatic, and the two of us sat up in a beautiful Tiger Moth — helmets on, open cockpit — and took off from Mascot, which was not much more than a grassy paddock at the time.

Two years later, Keith and I were again at Mascot together, along with 300,000 other well-wishers, welcoming home Charles

Kingsford Smith and his magnificent *Southern Cross* after his historic flight across the Pacific. Kingsford Smith captured our young imaginations like no other. He was my boyhood hero who, combined with the memory of my father's travel tales, reinforced in me that there was a whole lot of world out there just waiting to be explored.

THE WORLD I KNEW as a child was one of courtesy and obedience, where manners and modesty were mandatory. I was indoctrinated with the belief that in life you get back what you put in. If you had a problem, it was up to you to find a solution and rise above it. Making public your personal feelings was not done and sons did not cry. These were very different times: individual gripes did not sit well in comparison to memories of the First World War and surviving the Depression. How we felt about things wasn't the main priority and there was certainly no such thing as counselling. It was a world of rules that children were expected to learn and respect: don't speak unless spoken to; honour commitments; always arrive on time; never outstay your welcome; close doors quietly; no whingeing — the list was ever-growing. It was also a time when a very little went a long way. Being frugal was an art form every family learned how to perfect. Once a week my mother cooked a roast and my father would carve the meat prudently, ensuring there would be enough left over to use in meals over the following days.

Despite all this, I remember feeling as though I was living in very exciting times. During the late 1920s, Australia, it seemed to me, was on the cusp of technological change, and I was fascinated. I had always been a boldly curious child. If I received a toy I dismantled it on day one to find out how it worked and then I'd put it back together again. I had to understand how things worked. I was known for quite a while as 'Little Why', because I would ask a question and before anyone had time to finish explaining it to me, I'd pipe up with 'But why?' My mind was always teeming with unanswered questions. I relished the challenge of putting things together — model airplanes in particular. The model kits were made of balsa, a light wood, and I took great pains to piece the planes together with precision. My parents encouraged my activities, partitioning one end of the back veranda of our house and allocating it as 'Rowley's corner'. It was in this corner where I kept my precious belongings — the odd toy or bits and pieces I collected from around the neighbourhood with which to build things. I was a bower bird even then.

My father further fuelled my interest in all things technical and scientific when he introduced me to my first crystal wireless set. One of his workmates was a real crank with wireless sets and my father asked him to make one for me when I was about twelve. No one we knew could afford to buy a licensed radio receiver from a shop and there was little need: amateurs all over the country were busy tinkering in back sheds, making their own crystal sets. Mine consisted of two cylinders wound with fine copper wire and a crystal with a 'cat's whisker' — a piece of fine wire. I pressed the cat's whisker onto a sensitive point on the crystal to pick up the radio signal, which I listened to through a homemade headset. I relayed to my father and mother what was being broadcast so they could share in the experience. The crackling voices of strangers coming from somewhere out in the ether was the most incredible thing in the world to me at the time. The relatively quiet world I knew was becoming louder, and I couldn't get enough of it.

Powerful man-made machines were being invented and monumental projects were being undertaken: the railway system was becoming progressively electrified across the city and the world of aviation captivated young boys everywhere. I loved the sound of Gipsy Moth aircraft buzzing over the city; I craned my neck skywards every time I heard one coming. Nothing took hold of our imaginations more, though, than the building of the Sydney Harbour Bridge. Keith and I were infatuated with its development (as was, no doubt, every other boy in Sydney at the time). Occasionally we travelled by train and tram into the city to check on its progress, but we mainly kept track from the newspaper reports — trips to town were a rare and expensive treat. We did, however, attend the opening of the workshops at Milson's Point. We found it absolutely mind-boggling to view all the heavy machinery, and attempting to wrap our science-crazy brains around the process of how they were building this landmark structure only heightened our fixation. Keith and I were each given a heavy rivet from one of the workshops as a souvenir; I still have mine to this day. I remember clearly the pylons emerging first and then the incredible sprouting of the northern and southern arches, which appeared suspended in space until they were joined in 1929.

Through the Depression, too, technology represented progress and we clung to progress as a harbinger of better times. Man seemed to be moving ahead at a frenetic pace and we hoped that a new and thrilling way of life would be waiting for us at the end of the economic slump. It was only a matter of time.

AT THE BEGINNING OF my adolescence I was introduced to a new way of life: country life. My Aunt Linda had met and married a doctor, Arthur Lewis, in 1926, and the pair had immediately moved to Kyogle on the north coast of New South Wales. I made my first visit there when aged twelve. My parents couldn't afford to come with me but I had access to a concession train pass and they were happy for me to enjoy all of my school holidays with Linda and Arthur. By around 1930, my brother Frank had moved to Kyogle to live with Linda and Arthur permanently. He had always been a sick child, suffering from chronic bronchial trouble. My parents thought he would be far better off living in the clean country air with a doctor in the house to help care for him.

Linda and Arthur lived in the township in a big house on a large block. They had an enormous veranda, about three metres wide and 25 metres long, and a large rose garden that extended right down to a back paddock which fronted the next street. It was this back paddock that was of most interest to me, because this was where the horses were kept. I was very fortunate to have access to a beautiful riding and sulky pony called Sally. One of Arthur's grateful patients who was moving from the district had given it to him for us kids to ride. She was about fourteen hands in size with a lovely dark roan coat. Horse riding was a big drawcard, along with spending time with my baby cousin Margaret ('Pat'), who was eleven years my junior and like a sister to me.

I made plenty of friends in Kyogle. I didn't spend a lot of time with my brother: we were as chalk and cheese, and had very different friends. I had two great mates in particular: Duncan McNaughton and Des Makepeace. Duncan was the 'butcher boy', a delivery boy. He rode his horse around town taking deliveries of meat to various houses. The butcher, Cyril Croker, had a couple of horses for his butcher boys, and he used to let me ride one of them before I had access to Sally. Des was the son of the local bank manager. Linda and Arthur often used to go on picnics with the Makepeaces and that's how Des and I became friends. Des's father developed appendicitis and died of peritonitis when we were in our early teens. When Des and his mother had to leave Kyogle, Linda arranged for them to live with my grandparents in Gower Street, and my Kyogle friend quickly became my Summer Hill friend — and ultimately one of my lifelong closest mates.

Far from my mother's rules of propriety, Kyogle gave me the opportunity to misbehave. I would often round up a group of local kids — ensuring we included the police sergeant's daughter, just in case we were booked for something — and ride out to one of the many properties where farmers grew melons in between their corn crops. We loved to split open enormous watermelons and have a great feed; face first into the pink flesh, we stuffed ourselves to near bursting point. Then we climbed back on our horses and let them gallop at their own will, watermelon sloshing in our bellies. We often made ourselves sick, but that was part of the fun.

My visits to Kyogle also proved to be invaluable work experience. A great treat was to accompany Arthur on his rounds. Being 'on rounds' made me feel very grown up and another step closer to becoming a doctor, even though I was only waiting in the front seat of his car on the majority of visits.

I loved so many things about my trips to the country, particularly the opportunity to 'go bush'. Each year I used to go out with the tick inspectors, riding on Sally. They filled dips with water and anti-tick poison, and then they'd run the cattle through. I would help the inspectors and the owners round up the cattle. If some of the herd broke away down a hill, the inspectors and farm boys would go screaming off after them, but big brave me used to go round the long way; there was no way I was going to break my neck going down a hill. I spent a fair amount of time watching these bushies at work because they fascinated me. These men could mend any old thing with a bit of fencing wire, a pair of pliers and an innate ability to improvise. On other occasions, I was invited to go out with bullock teams to the McPherson Ranges, north of the border town of Cougal, some 50 kilometres from Kyogle. Whenever I had the chance, I'd take off from the team to go exploring in the rainforest on my own. Those mountain ponies were magnificent and sure-footed; they really knew the terrain. It was extraordinarily beautiful and very rugged country — as rugged as the teak forests I would one day come to know in Burma.

CHAPTER TWO

AUSTRALIA AT WAR

When I was accepted as a student at Fort Street Boys' High School, a selective school in the inner Sydney suburb of Petersham, I really got my comeuppance. I had been a reasonably good scholar up until then, always in the top handful of students in intermediate high school, but I quickly discovered there were much bigger academic fish in the Fort Street pond. I could rattle off algebraic formulae but my rote memory was poor: I was far from being the teacher's pet in history or languages. Forced to read Shakespeare, I resented being told to spend hours hunting for hidden meanings in words and phrases which, at the time, I was convinced Shakespeare had never intended.

I was young, impatient and had also developed a deep fear of failure. I did not like what I was not good at, and I attempted to control my fear by avoiding any field of activity in which I did not believe I had a reasonable chance of success. I stuck to science and maths, where I felt safe. Outside the classroom, I suspected I would be hopeless at football and cricket, so I never tried. I played tennis instead, at which I was not brilliant, but neither were the friends I played against, and that was what mattered. I always aimed to be as good as or better than my peers — so I made sure I selected my friends carefully. Looking back, I can see the link between my fear of failure and my childhood experiences of prejudice. My fears propelled me in my determination to prove that I could match it with anyone else I came up against in life — friend or foe.

I can now contemplate certain events of my adolescence as veiled preparation for the circumstances I would experience later in life. Hindsight is a wonderful thing; it allows you to draw connections between events in your life that were a mystery to you at the time. I clearly recall becoming quite self-conscious about my appearance when I started high school. I wore glasses and was still very chubby — I had a round face, a tubby tummy, arms and legs — just like my mother, and I vowed I would not end up like her, puffing and panting as she played each shot on our tennis court. So I simply stopped eating as much and slimmed down quite quickly. During the Depression, it was hardly a challenge: I just cut back on bread and dripping. My parents thought my weight loss was probably just part of being a teenager; they were not aware that I had made a deliberate decision to become unconcerned by food. I adopted the ethos of 'eat to live, don't live to eat'. It wasn't until I became a prisoner of war, when all around me men were dropping dead from malnutrition and disease, that I would really come to appreciate the immeasurable value of this decision — but that story is still to come.

My closest friends were Des Makepeace, my Kyogle friend who had moved to Sydney, and Syd Smith, whom I met through Des. After school we spent as much time together as our parents would allow, while in the classroom I put my head down and worked furiously to keep pace with my fellow Fort Street students. My goal of studying medicine remained at the forefront of my competitive mind, further encouraged by Arthur Lewis during my ongoing visits to Kyogle during holiday periods.

Midway through my final year of high school I started making plans, ever so discreetly, to become an actuary — just in case I failed to matriculate into medicine. I wasn't retreating from what I really wanted, but rather ensuring I could withdraw to a position of strength via an honourable exit strategy, so I wouldn't be seen as a flop. Thankfully, my contingency plan became redundant when I matriculated in 1933 and was accepted into the medical school at the University of Sydney. I was significantly relieved, but didn't let it show.

I had no way of paying my way through university, but I didn't let this concern me too greatly; after all, my parents had drummed into me that every problem has a solution, so I found one. I took out a life insurance policy, nominating Arthur as the beneficiary, and he kindly loaned me the money I needed. I was seventeen years old and on my way to becoming a doctor.

MY INTRODUCTION TO MILITARY life coincided with the beginning of my medical studies. Within weeks of classes commencing, many of my fellow students were joining the Sydney University Regiment — part of the Militia but with membership confined to students only. I hesitated to follow suit: the prospect of spending all my waking hours with peers either in class or at the University Regiment was not appealing. The regular Militia (today known as the Army Reserve), which anyone was free to join, and where I knew I would meet a broad range of people, seemed a much more agreeable choice. I also noticed that members of the University Regiment seemed to see themselves as more elite than those in the regular Militia. Perhaps my uneasiness with this type of superiority also influenced my decision, but above all else I just wanted to stick with my good friends Des and Syd, who had already joined the 1st Artillery Survey Company in the regular Militia.

I was only seventeen when I decided to sign up, two months short of the minimum age for enlisting. The Militia was more than keen for new recruits, so no one bothered to question my youthful looks when I declared I was eighteen. Back then, most young men felt a sense of loyalty to the 'old country' and, having grown up in the wake of the First World War, we believed it was our duty to join one of the services. Arthur had served in the First World War and several of my mother's ancestors had been members of the Royal Navy so, for me, it was also a matter of family tradition. Thoughts of a real war did not cross my mind. It was 1934 and the Second World War was still five years away.

The fact that a lot of maths was involved in the Artillery Survey Company pleased me no end. The company was divided into three sections: Surveying, Flash Spotting and Sound Ranging. The Surveying Section, responsible for pure surveying, fixed trig points to establish the coordinates of major features in our area. The Flash Spotting Section observed the 'flash' of an enemy gun while looking through a surveying instrument called a director (similar to a theodolite); they measured the angle between the flash and a previously established point of reference to determine the position of an enemy gun. The Sound Ranging Section planted microphones out in the field, in predetermined surveyed positions, in a perfectly straight line. Because sound travels in waves, the sound of a gun would reach the nearest microphone first, and then there would be a time-lag before it reached the next one, and so on. Then it was purely a case of plotting the position of an enemy gun from the time intervals recorded. For my scientific brain, this was bliss.

I joined the 1st Artillery Survey Company at the lowly rank of gunner. It was my job to help lay the wires to each of the microphones in the Sound Ranging Section. The double-copper wires, thick and heavy, were wound around huge wooden reels. Working with a partner, I had to place a steel rod through a reel and drag it along to run out the wire; it was incredibly heavy work. My back and arms ached for days after each session.

We were required to attend a weekly parade at Victoria Barracks, as well as occasional weekend bivouacs and an annual two-week training camp. I balanced my time carefully between university and Militia commitments, while Des studied accountancy and Syd worked for an insurance company. At the conclusion of our weekly parades, we would walk together, three abreast, to Central Station. Des and Syd, both a good few inches taller than me, loved to sidle up to me, one on either side, and then lift me off the ground, holding me by an elbow each. They thought it was a great trick to play on their much shorter mate.

My first three years of medicine were spent on campus studying physiology, anatomy and biochemistry. In 1937 I commenced my fourth year at St Vincent's Public Hospital in Darlinghurst, where I found myself surrounded by the Catholics my grandfather had warned me to avoid. As a child, I remember wondering how my grandfather knew who was a Catholic — they always looked the same as Protestants to me — and now I knew for certain that they were. For years 4, 5 and 6 of the course we spent our mornings at the medical school and our afternoons at the hospital. Every day on the wards we learned something new: how to take histories, examine a patient, and recognise the normal and then the abnormal. It was all very exciting coming into contact with real patients and observing and recording real cases. Nothing surprised me; I have always felt at home in a hospital. There were no clichéd fainting episodes from shock, or days when I wanted to quit. I was gripped by medicine from day one. Ever keen to impress my patients, I wore my shiny stethoscope like a badge of honour.

I found light relief from study in the form of poker, which I played with Mick Ireland, a friend from university. Mick lived in Strathfield and was the proud owner of a wonderful 'Baby' Austin car. He often picked me up from Summer Hill on his way to university. We played 'penny poker' in between lectures, logging whatever we won or lost at the end of each session in a little black book. At the end of the week we tallied our figures and, more often than not, we broke even, which was lucky for me considering my limited finances.

I continued to spend holidays with Arthur and Linda at Kyogle. Since beginning university, Arthur had allowed me to assist in the operating theatre. In city theatres, there was usually a surgeon, an assisting surgeon, and then two or three others trying to get into the act. The assistants would swab and retract as directed, or cut the stitches, that kind of thing — boring as hell, but a help to the surgeon nonetheless. In a country town, a surgeon didn't have the luxury of an assisting surgeon, let alone a whole team, so Arthur developed techniques that allowed him to do most things himself or with limited assistance. He taught me operating techniques that ensured minimum trauma for the patient. He showed me how to remove an appendix, for example, through a very small incision. Many of the city surgeons I observed made incisions eight or nine centimetres long; I used to watch some of them put their hand right inside a patient's abdomen and feel around to find the appendix. Whereas Arthur, by careful history taking and thorough examinations prior to the operation, only needed to make an incision less than three centimetres in length and could then pull the appendix out with one finger, two at the most. That he happened to be ambidextrous was also very convenient: he could snip or stitch with either hand. He instructed me to take notes during every operation I witnessed, very specific notes — to the point of knowing how often the patient coughed or exactly when his or her eye twitched. I walked out of each operation with a handwritten screed from which to study and learn. I still have my notes from some of the operations I assisted with at Kyogle.

The matron at Kyogle Memorial Hospital was Nora McKidd. She told me I had to learn about theatre from the ground up, literally, and ordered me to scrub the walls and floors of the theatre. 'Until it's *spotless*,' she said. Matron McKidd was a big-chested woman, built like an operatic soprano. Her uniform was always gleaming white and crisply starched. In my early days as a medical student, she had appointed me as the 'dirty nurse', a position at the very bottom of the theatre's pecking order. It was my job to remove the bucket of blood-and-bits from the theatre after each operation and dispose of it. Matron McKidd was one of the old brigade, a stickler for procedure and discipline but with a kind heart.

The long holiday periods I spent at Kyogle were seminal days. Matron McKidd drilled me in the importance of hygiene, while Arthur taught me to observe, record and analyse — the basic tenets of the scientific method. He also taught me that, as a surgeon, you need to make every movement count; it should only take minimal movement to achieve whatever it is you need to achieve.

WHILE I HAD BEEN enjoying a relatively carefree life between Summer Hill and trips to Kyogle, I remained conscious of the world in turmoil. I had followed in the newspapers the Japanese invasion of China in 1937 and vaguely recall thinking that this might have been a precursor to war, but I don't remember feeling anxious about another world war approaching. The world had certainly been changing throughout the 1930s. I was taking notice, keeping up with the news like everyone else, but mostly I was absorbed in my own life of medical studies and socialising. By late August in 1939, however, Australians were acutely aware of Hitler's ever-increasing military aggression and his demands on Poland; it seemed almost inevitable that Britain would soon declare war, and that Australia would follow. War was unquestionably upon us.

In the last week of August I was contacted by the officer commanding the 1st Artillery Survey Company, Major Len Heerey. He advised that I had passed my exams to become a lieutenant in the Militia, and would soon be officially gazetted, meaning my name would be listed in the official *Government Gazette*. I had been determined to rise through Militia ranks as quickly as I could. Since joining in 1934 I had passed the exams for promotion from gunner to lance bombardier, bombardier and then sergeant. Heerey referred me to his military tailor so I could have a uniform made before I was due to commence training at a camp in Dapto, on the south coast of New South Wales, the following weekend. At that particular moment I thought the King and I were about equal in status.

The night before I was due at Dapto, I took Barbara Blazey, a favourite girl of mine at the time, to Manly. We caught the ferry across Sydney Harbour and then walked along the wharf, arm in arm. Neither of us talked much, we remained deep in our own thoughts of what the war might mean to us and our families, as well as to the country. It was officially the end of party time; life was about to become a whole lot more earnest. I remember the pavement was covered in sheets of newsprint flapping in the evening breeze. People were snatching late edition newspapers from news stands just to read the headlines — 'War Imminent', 'Threat of War' — and then tossing them aside. I distinctly recall not feeling any fear about the onset of war; I accepted it as inevitable and, on reflection, even with a naïve sense of anticipation. Australia was not under any direct threat and we were only going to war to help our mother country, not defend our own — or so we thought at the time.

I arrived at Dapto the following day, 3 September, complete with the one pip of a second lieutenant on my new officer's uniform. The three officers senior to me had enlisted in the Second Australian Imperial Force overnight, and I suddenly found myself, at age 23, as officer commanding the Sound Ranging Group.

On that first night in camp, we were settling down in the officers' mess after dinner when we heard Prime Minister Robert

Menzies announce over the airwaves the news we had been expecting: 'It is my melancholy duty to inform you, officially, that in consequence of a persistence by Germany and her invasion of Poland, Great Britain has declared war upon her, and that as a result Australia is also at war.'

The younger ones of our company, me included, were high spirited and animated in our enthusiasm. At last, we thought, we would have the opportunity to do what we had been training to do for years now. Heerey, a quiet and efficient man, quickly took control of his men; there were procedures to follow. Inside a safe situated at camp headquarters sat two revolvers and a large envelope marked 'Secret', which contained our orders. Heerey calmly ordered the adjutant to fetch the envelope and then opened it without delay. I don't remember what our orders were, but I do recall our initial zeal becoming increasingly suppressed as Heerey spoke. I can also recall the reaction of the older men amongst us, veterans of the First World War. They were silent; their minds no doubt boiling with memories of what war was really about — and what the rest of us were still to learn the hard way.

BY THE END OF 1939, with my final medical exams out of the way, I set myself the objective of joining the Second Australian Imperial Force (AIF). Australia, in effect, had two armies: the Militia, responsible for home defence and confined to Australia, and the AIF, a volunteer force eligible for overseas service and responsible for imperial defence requirements. I viewed the AIF as a natural progression after six years' training in the Militia. Many of us felt that the First World War was still unfinished business, that Germany was never truly defeated and had always remained an active enemy. I didn't glorify war but there was definitely an element of it that appealed to my boyhood spirit of adventure. Some might find the simplicity of my motivation to enlist difficult to comprehend. Countless times I have been asked: but after the First World War, how could you have been blind to the risks you were taking? The answer is uncomplicated. We were not blind to the risks — I did not deny death as a possibility, but in my raw and youthful enthusiasm I just hoped it would be some other poor buggers, rather than me, who might not make it home again.

On passing my final medical exams I commenced my residency at the Mater Misericordiae Hospital in North Sydney. I was impatient to enlist in the AIF, but realised I needed to complete my hospital training if I wanted to officially claim to be of use as a doctor. I remained in the Militia during 1940, attending further camps in the Maitland area of New South Wales and making the most of my learning time at the Mater, but always looking forward to my move out into the big wide world.

Throughout my years in the Militia, I had come to know quite a few men who held senior Army positions, one of whom was Brigadier Cecil 'Boots' Callaghan, Commander of the Royal Australian Artillery (RAA). He owned a boot and shoe store in George Street in the city and, not surprisingly, he was a fanatic about polished leather boots. He regarded being neatly turned out as more important than remembering your rifle. Boots knew I was anxious to join the AIF; I had spoken to him about it on previous occasions, and he was also aware I had my heart set on going into an artillery unit as a regimental medical officer (RMO). So when he contacted me in late August to suggest it might be a good time to consider enlisting, I didn't hesitate. I knew he had enough seniority at Division Headquarters to arrange something for me. Strictly speaking, I should have waited until the end of the year, when I would have officially completed my residency, but I figured if I counted the numerous operations Arthur had allowed me to perform at Kyogle over the past few years, then surely I had exceeded all requirements.

On 2 September 1940, I left the Militia to join the AIF. Upon enlistment at the Sydney Agricultural Showground at Moore

Park (today known as Fox Studios) I became a captain, with three proud pips on my shoulder. Most of the medical officers enlisting in the AIF had no previous military experience, so training in Army procedures and drills were, for them, compulsory, while for the majority of Militia men we spent the following days partying with friends and filling in time, awaiting further orders. The war was a very serious business, but the reality of what we were getting ourselves into hadn't yet pierced the surface of our brash egos. We were competitive among ourselves, eager to prove to fresh recruits — especially those without any Militia training — that we knew what we were on about. Only a couple of days after enlisting in the AIF we were carrying on like old hands, greeting new and bewildered young recruits at the gates with a smug 'You'll be sorry.'

After four days at the showground I was posted to a Militia unit that was in need of an RMO. I was very conscious of being given a Militia posting when I had just become part of the AIF (rudely unaware that I was showing a glimpse of the same prejudice I had always loathed in others!), but the unofficial arrangement, via Boots, was that I should remain with the Militia unit until another AIF artillery unit was formed. I just had to be patient.

The Militia unit was training at the old Liverpool camp in south-west Sydney. The camp, originally built during 1914, had been occupied by the AIF during the Great War. Inside the huts, straw stuffing from old mattresses had fallen through wide cracks between the floorboards. Over time, straw and dust had accumulated to form a solid rotting mass beneath the well-worn floors. I organised the men to clean out the area beneath the huts in an attempt to control an epidemic of respiratory infection. Tonnes of refuse were removed. Initially, the men were resistant, but they changed their minds when they discovered that along with the straw many coins had also fallen through the gaping floorboards. The return on a daily basis varied between several shillings up to a few pounds.

Thanks to the influence of Kyogle's Matron McKidd, I was unrelenting in my insistence on hygiene within the camp. We cleaned up garbage that had been pitched from the camp area over the riverbank, and focused on fly control. The not-so-good-humoured men in my unit voted me top of their 'shark list' — declaring they would feed me to the sharks if we were ever on convoy overseas together. On reflection, I admit that I was a cocky little bugger — I still had much to learn in the art of man management. Fortunately for me I would soon encounter great leaders from whom I could learn.

ON 10 NOVEMBER, TWO months into my time at Liverpool, I received word to contact Boots at Division Headquarters. I was delighted to hear his voice. He advised that the 27th Brigade had been raised together with the 2/15th Field Regiment to which it was attached.[1] I was to be RMO of the 2/15th Field Regiment, under the command of Lieutenant Colonel John O'Neill. Boots gave me the telephone number for the new regiment. 'Call Colonel O'Neill for instructions. Congratulations and good luck,' he said, before hanging up the phone.

I was elated: the old boy had honoured his promise. Finally I was going to serve as a real soldier — and I couldn't wait.

CHAPTER THREE

BOUND FOR ACTION

After my conversation with Boots, I promptly called my new regiment and asked to speak to Lieutenant Colonel John O'Neill. 'There is no 2/15th Field Regiment. There is no Colonel O'Neill,' came the reply. I had been involved with the military for long enough to suspect this was probably standard security procedure; I waited in silence, listening to whispering voices at the end of the line. Having decided I was not a spy, the voice told me to report to O'Neill at Rosebery Racecourse the following day.

So early on the morning of 11 November, I left Liverpool camp in a borrowed staff car with driver, bound for the headquarters of my new AIF regiment. I was jubilant at the thought of serving under O'Neill, whom I had first met during my Militia days. I knew him to be a very competent gunner and a born leader of men: whenever he spoke, it was clear he was in command. He looked his men in the eye and made them feel valued. He had a cheery face with black bushy eyebrows and a neatly trimmed Chaplinesque moustache. Like Boots, he was fastidious about his men being neatly turned out. Upon arrival at the racecourse, I presented myself all spit and polish to O'Neill. He greeted me warmly. 'Richards,' he said, shaking my freckled hand. 'Delighted to have a gunner officer as our RMO. Welcome.'

To be acknowledged as a gunner (an artilleryman as distinct from the rank of gunner) filled me with pride. There is a well-known saying among artillerymen: 'Once a gunner, always a gunner', and while I had officially converted from the artillery to the medical corps upon enlisting in the AIF, I only ever considered myself as a gunner who happened to be performing a medical job. Unless you have been in the military, it will be difficult to understand the significance of belonging to an artillery unit. It goes back to the early days of horse-drawn gun crews, where each member had to pull his weight, even the horses, and the whole crew depended on one another. Each man was an essential link in a chain that bound the unit together — one of the greatest fears an artilleryman entertained was that he might let his team-mates down. As gunners, we learnt to recognise and respect the weaknesses and strengths of our team members while basking in the development of brotherly love, understanding and kindness. Once you were a gunner, you never forgot that you were serving in a unit where fierce loyalty was essential, and respect was a currency you had genuinely earned. When I became an artilleryman, I knew I was matching it with the best, and that the foundations of true mateship were being laid.

O'Neill introduced me to Major Jack Meyers and Major Frank Ball, the battery commanders, and to Lieutenant Theo LeMaistre Walker, the intelligence officer. All three men had served in the Militia in field artillery and were now going through the transition from horse-drawn guns to mechanised units. Technology was changing warfare even then.

'Move into camp at Ingleburn on 15 November. Call on the adjutant for movement orders,' O'Neill instructed. 'I'll see you there.'

'Yes, sir,' I replied, before being dismissed.

Feeling on top of the world, I climbed back into my borrowed car for the return trip to Liverpool. While driving along Oxford Street, towards the city, I noticed that the traffic was exceptionally heavy. Impatient, I asked the driver to duck down a side street, only to discover that it, too, was congested; in fact, all cars were at a standstill. The streets were silent. My driver turned around to face me in the back seat. His face was solemn. 'Sir,' he said, 'today is the eleventh of November — and it's the eleventh hour.'

I lowered my head in shame. In my great excitement I had forgotten it was Armistice Day. I sat to attention to observe the two minutes' silence.

AS ORDERED, I JOINED the founding officers of the 2/15th Field Regiment at Ingleburn, where I was allocated a hut at the end of the camp as my regimental aid post (RAP). Covered in dust and rubbish, it had clearly been unoccupied for some time. I was in the midst of surveying the mess when I heard a soft voice. 'Excuse me, sir, are you the RMO?' A grey-haired soldier was standing at the door, looking bewildered and a little sheepish.

I replied in the affirmative and he quickly announced himself as Corporal Jim Armstrong, who was to be my medical orderly. He looked uncomfortable in his uniform; he wore his hat rather square instead of on an angle. He was a tall, heavily built man and I couldn't help but notice his hands: they were huge. I introduced him to what was to be our RAP, told him it needed to be tidied up and then left him to it.

A couple of hours later I returned to find that everything had been thoroughly scrubbed: the floor, the table tops, even the legs of the tables. The hut looked spanking new. Jim had set up the office with chairs and benches, and on the table, which he had covered neatly with a blanket, sat a big wicker pannier with a large Red Cross on top. Whoever this man was, he certainly wasn't afraid of hard work. It marked the beginning of a long and meaningful medical partnership. Within our regiment Jim became known as 'Old Silver', a term of endearment owing to his prematurely grey hair, while I was dubbed the 'Baby Doctor', thanks to my boyish appearance.

By mid-December, our regiment had received all of its drafts, including one Lieutenant Des Makepeace. My other closest friend, Syd Smith, had also gained a commission and enlisted in the 7th Division, bound for the Middle East. I was not surprised to see Des; I had helped arrange his recruitment when I heard that one of my fellow officers was looking for a survey officer. The moment Des arrived in camp we shot each other a knowing glance and grin: mission accomplished.

The regiment by this time had most of the equipment it needed, together with 18-pounder guns — *real* guns. We were just settling in to function as a unit when we received orders to move to the Manoeuvre Paddock, outside the School of Artillery at Holdsworthy. I'm still unsure as to why we were ordered to move, perhaps Ingleburn was needed for the accommodation of infantry units, but regardless the men blamed every decision on the 'bastards from Army or Division Headquarters'. This was nothing new, and no different from the traditional 'workers versus the boss' division you come across in most workplaces — only in our case there was never any scope for right of reply. The move was to be effected by 1 January and Des and I, known for our Militia surveying experience, were sent on a reconnaissance mission.

Most of the proposed camp area was choked with shrubs, all of which needed to be cleared: it was no more than an overgrown paddock. During the following days we planned and surveyed a storm water drainage system and the general layout of the camp with the assistance of Captain Clive Walker, a surveyor in civilian life. Following a curtailed Christmas dinner with my family in Summer Hill, Des and I returned to camp to finish planning for the move. There was a job to be done and we wanted to get on with it.

On Boxing Day, along with an advance party of workers, we put our plans into action. The camp area was cleared with heavy chains slung between two gun tractors. We pegged out various drains, paths, tent lines, mess lines and kitchens. We installed a very effective drainage system for storm water, as well as effluent drains from the improvised fly-proofed kitchens and the ablution areas — complete with absorption pits and evaporation trenches. The food storehouse featured double walls made from green brush to keep the inside temperature cool and enable air to circulate. Some of the men in the advance work party had previously been in the Militia, where many had developed the useful art of 'acquiring' goods. We didn't bother questioning the origin of galvanised iron, chicken wire and other items not available through our normal quartermaster stores. After all, there was a war on, and we figured that the locals who suffered such losses were making their contribution (admittedly uninvited and unknowingly) to the military effort.

By the time the rest of our men moved from Ingleburn to Holdsworthy on 4 January, large white tents had been erected in rows, and the camp became known as 'Tent Town', attracting attention in the *Sydney Morning Herald*:

AIF BUILDS OWN HOME:
Camp in bush is model

In little more than a week, young artillerymen have converted a wilderness of scrub on the outskirts of Holdsworthy into a model camp which has amazed experienced Army officers.

So far as is known, it is the first time that an AIF unit in training in New South Wales, starting from 'scratch', has built its own home.

So well have the men carried out their task that officers say it would 'break their hearts' if they had to move from the camp, which originally had been intended only as temporary quarters . . .

— January 1941

Establishing the camp at Holdsworthy was our regiment's first significant team achievement, and we were peacock proud. All of us grew in confidence, convinced that we were becoming real soldiers very quickly; already we felt unaccountably brave. When I think back now, I am somewhat surprised by the supreme self-confidence I possessed at the time. Some could certainly argue that I was overconfident: straight out of medical school and in charge of the health and wellbeing of a regiment of men, a huge responsibility — but I was fearless. I didn't doubt myself for a second. Arthur had trained me to be a self-contained doctor, not to rely on medical teams for support, and I can honestly say that I felt I had enough military training and medical knowledge to cope with the responsibilities ahead. In my mind, my role as RMO was not daunting but rather a reward, my just desserts for years of dedicated training, study and practical experience. I thought I was ready for anything — but no amount of buoyant confidence could have ever prepared any of us for the horrors in the years ahead.

Even with the considerable training load, including gun drills, signalling, gun-tractor driving, hygiene and first aid, many still found time and energy to 'play'. Some went AWL (absent without leave) at night, but providing they were back on deck at reveille little was said or done about it. O'Neill, nicknamed 'Peggy', was an extremely good judge of men; he earned the respect and later the affection of his troops because of his fairness, tolerance and strict maintenance of morale and discipline without the usual use of the charge sheet and orderly room. One example stands out in my mind above all others. Early in the piece, a young and inexperienced soldier wrote home to his mother about some of the men playing two-up in the Salvation Army marquee. Disgusted, his mother promptly wrote to her local member of parliament, who passed on the complaint to the Minister of the Army, who then sent a rocket via RAA Headquarters to O'Neill. His own response was far from that of a conventional AIF commanding officer (CO). At the end of an evening mess, he quietly called upon Stuart Ward, the adjutant, and me to accompany him on a visit to the marquee in question.

A well-attended and noisy game of two-up was in full swing when we arrived and O'Neill immediately joined in. The men roared, endorsing the participation of their commanding officer in a forbidden game. After losing his own money, O'Neill borrowed from Ward and me until his luck changed. Having had his early education in the pool rooms of Melbourne, he soon had a pile of cash in front of him. Following a few more tosses, O'Neill pushed his winnings towards the senior sergeant present. 'Please give the sergeants' mess president my compliments, and convert these winnings into beer for the men,' he said. The rowdy mob started cheering again and O'Neill, Ward and I got up to leave.

Before departing, O'Neill stood tall in front of his men and added: 'And *never* again let me catch you playing two-up.'

We left the men in silence — dead silence — and never again did we hear of two-up being played in the Salvation Army marquee. The men obviously made more discreet arrangements; they wouldn't dare let Peggy down. O'Neill had only further enhanced his authority, and he had lost no respect in the process.

AMIDST MOUNTING CONCERN OVER the security of Singapore, long considered an 'impregnable fortress', and increasing tensions in the Pacific, Australia's War Cabinet had offered a brigade of the 8th Division AIF to British Prime Minister Winston Churchill in

December 1940. Singapore, with Hong Kong to the north, India to the west and Australia and New Zealand to the south-east, had long been seen as a vital defence point for imperial security.[1] The majority of Australians assumed that Singapore provided a guarantee of protection for their own homeland. By early January 1941, the 22nd Brigade and its supporting units had sailed out of Sydney on the *Queen Mary*, bound for the British colony of Malaya. While officially we did not know where our regiment would be sent, the odds seemed likely we would soon join the 22nd Brigade in Malaya — and that our probable enemy would be Japan. We had long expected our adversary to be Germany, but it made little difference. We had been trained to be prepared for 'the enemy', and wherever that enemy came from didn't change how we felt about going to war. Amongst our men there was the feeling of 'it will be our turn soon', and our feet were itching.

I had never seen a tropical jungle before but I imagined parts of Malaya to be like the subtropical rainforest I used to ride through at Cougal, near Kyogle: hot, humid and dense with towering pea-green trees and a shaded forest floor. With the prospect of jungle warfare now firmly fixed in our minds, O'Neill and I anticipated our regiment might be widely dispersed during action, and that the control of malaria, dysentery and skin diseases would be the most significant medical problems. After attending a course at the School of Hygiene and Tropical Medicine at the Sydney Agricultural Showground in late January, I returned to camp eager to share my knowledge. I devised a medical prevention strategy and put it to O'Neill that it would be wise to have not only well-trained hygiene people throughout our regiment, but also a number of trained first aiders. Back in my Militia days, I had been introduced to Captain John Loewenthal, RMO of the 2/9th Field Regiment. Loewenthal had trained and appointed two of his gunners to be battery medical orderlies — which was not standard Army procedure. I thought having additional men medically trained was a damned good idea, but why stop at training only two extra men? So I expanded the concept.

With O'Neill's support, a five-day first-aid and nursing course was planned. Despite strong objections from the battery commanders, who wanted all men on artillery training, 67 men were selected to participate in the course to ensure the widest possible distribution of first-aid skills throughout our regiment. The course covered St John Ambulance first aid, Army field ambulance training, and nursing, including the management of simulated casualties. I invited nurses from a nearby medical unit to participate in the training, to add interest and boost our attendance rate. For the most interested students, we conducted advanced training at the RAP, and from the best of these we selected battery and troop medical orderlies.[2]

The troop medical orderlies were responsible for daily skin inspections of the men in their respective troops. I trained them to check for rashes, abrasions, lacerations, tinea and early signs of ulcers; to treat minor conditions and send the more serious cases to the RAP at the earliest instance. These men became extremely competent and, in days to come, would prove to be worth their weight in gold.

My priority was the prevention of illness and injury, largely through strict hygiene and first-aid training, rather than solely concentrating on treatment. I was essentially trying to plan myself out of a job: if I could prevent illness and disease then I wouldn't be spending every waking hour treating my men and using valuable supplies during action. The philosophy of prevention, as obvious as it might now seem, was still quite unusual at the time — despite statistics from the First World War verifying that far more people had died from illness and disease compared to the number who died as a result of battle casualties. Back in Kyogle, Uncle Arthur was singularly appalled by my interest in hygiene.

He maintained that I had been trained to treat the sick and the wounded — not, as he said, 'to look up drains'. While he supported first-aid training, he considered matters of hygiene as 'the bottom of the dish' in terms of medical importance, and not the responsibility of an RMO. I disagreed: I viewed it as essential and directly related to my job of preventing illness and disease.

The additional first-aid training was unique to our regiment, which meant we needed extra money for medical supplies. An appeal over radio station 2UE provided finance to kit out each first aider with a haversack containing field dressings, bandages and other supplies which I trained them how to use. Each of the batteries and troops was also equipped with a felt-lined steel box with a canvas cover which contained enough equipment and supplies to run a makeshift RAP. Included in each box was a list of all items and a detailed guide to the use and dosage of all medications.

Not long after the training course was held, I was invited to a mess dinner at a camp in neighbouring Ingleburn. The dinner was in celebration of the completion of a month-long training camp by the Militia field ambulance, and was hosted by CO Lieutenant Colonel Pete Davies, whom I had known well during my Militia days. After generous hospitality, including several rounds of port, I asked Pete what was happening to his unused medical supplies and suggested I could make use of them. He was happy to order his quartermaster to let me have whatever I requested. The following morning I turned up in a truck and wiped out their shelves, leaving them with less than half of their supplies. I would later smuggle these same supplies into Birdwood Camp in Changi: they would prove to be an important lifeline in times when even a spoonful of rice would be considered a prized item.

Over the next few months, the intensity of training increased. The overall standard was set by O'Neill: he called the tune and the men followed willingly and with pride. Our men became skilled at handling their lusty 18-pounder guns and 4.5 howitzers. I continued to conduct hygiene drills and lectures. The men were initially somewhat resistant to my obsession with hygiene, but they followed orders. I know I got through to them: even today, whenever I find myself queuing in line at a buffet at a reunion or military function, almost unfailingly one of my men will come up behind me and say, 'Hey, Doc, have you sterilised that plate you're holding?'

While we continued to await our embarkation orders, I received word that two men from northern Malaya were visiting Sydney. Enthusiastic to learn as much as I could about our potential destination, I tracked these fellows down and invited them to our mess. Jim McNiven, a doctor, and Reg Nutt, a planter, both imparted lots of useful information on the prevention and management of skin problems, malaria and other tropical diseases. They made it clear that under no circumstances should we use ointment on skin; we should only use water-based creams or spirit-based lotions and paints. We learned that in the high humidity of the tropics, applying ointment would only serve to seal moisture on the skin — risking infection — whereas cream would dissolve. They also confirmed that the risk of tinea was high: they recommended that no man be allowed to walk anywhere without footwear, and that talcum powder be used sparingly to keep the skin dry. Such advice nowadays might seem trivial, but it was extremely important. Seemingly minor ailments could swiftly turn into tragedy: a fungal infection such as tinea could easily become infected with bacteria, immobilising entire units of men; and a tropical ulcer could result in amputation. Considering the majority of us had never before ventured outside Australia, we had little understanding of the problems associated with such a stinking hot and humid climate. I listened carefully, taking detailed and copious notes. I still had a lot to learn (even if I didn't always realise it at the time).

EMBARKATION ORDERS FINALLY ARRIVED on 12 July. We were granted leave two days later, and were due to depart Sydney by the end of the month: our destination was still not officially stated. The 6th, 7th and 9th Divisions AIF had so far been engaged in combat in the Mediterranean and North Africa. While early in the year Australia had enjoyed being part of morale-boosting Allied success against Italian forces in North Africa, it had been a very different and bloody story when they fought against the Germans in the Greece and Crete campaigns that followed in April and May. The consequences of these two latter engagements had been disastrous, with more than 5000 Australians taken as prisoners of war, almost 600 killed and hundreds wounded.[3] Despite these losses, Australia had continued to play an important part in the Allied invasion of Syria (an ally of the Vichy French government), and was persisting in its role of holding out against the forces of Germany's General Rommel in Tobruk. In comparison, the 8th Division — to which our regiment belonged — had been idle. We were almost relieved to be heading abroad at long last.

Some of our men remained hopeful we would be sent to the Middle East, where the real action was, while others were keen to join our fellow brigade in Malaya. I saw little point in having a preference — not knowing was simply part and parcel of military life: decisions from Army Headquarters were always enigmatic and it didn't much matter in a culture where you were expected to do as you were told anyway. We did not ask questions; we followed orders. Discipline was non-negotiable and there was no such thing as a committee decision: we were programmed to 'do or die'. Leaders were trained to make the decisions while the troops were trained to obey their leaders. We knew that everyone's lives could depend on the wrong action or the hesitation of just one man — and no one wanted to be that one man. We often argued about the pros and cons of decisions later, but never at the time an order was issued.

My parents had already resigned themselves to my departure and they were proud, as were my grandparents, our neighbours the Martins, and Arthur and Linda. The simple advice my mother offered the day before my departure was 'Come home soon.' My parents were stoic rather than emotional, maintaining their stiff upper lip. Thankfully, I did not have the added worry of leaving behind a special girlfriend: since joining the AIF I had been careful not to become too strongly attached to any of my girlfriends (and, let the record show, there were plenty!). I did not think it was fair to leave behind a fiancée when there was no guarantee we would return.

I saved my final farewell for my dear younger cousin Pat Lewis, with whom I had spent so much time during my visits to Kyogle. I had always been closer to Pat than my own brother. She was at boarding school in Pymble, so I made a special trip to the school on my final day of leave. She kindly presented me with a photo of herself. 'Carry it with you,' she said. Like my parents, Pat firmly believed she would see me again. 'Return it to me, in person, when you come home.'

I promised her I would do just that.

WE LEFT SYDNEY ON 29 July 1941 aboard the *Katoomba*, a luxury passenger ship. Early that morning we had moved from camp to Liverpool, where a train took us to Darling Harbour; the wheels of the train clacking loudly beneath our seats. Our movements were top secret but one of our men happened to be married to the stationmaster's daughter, so word spread amongst his friends about our estimated departure time. Their families and friends were waiting for them at Darling Harbour when we arrived, but for the majority of us — whose loved ones were not 'in the know' — our goodbyes were over.

Just prior to leaving Sydney, the men were hugely disappointed to discover that there would be no guns for the 2/15th Field

Regiment. Instead, we were issued with 3-inch mortars. After gruelling training on the guns up to a level of proud proficiency, the men were not impressed. However, with the knowledge that mortars (in the form of a short, thick tube and designed to fire a projectile at a steep angle) were well suited to being fired up and over tall trees in a jungle, the switch at least provided us with yet another clear sign we were indeed bound for Malaya.

It was a cool day, typical of late winter in Sydney when we sailed slowly down the harbour, passing beneath the beautiful bridge. The waters were dotted with several small craft all honking their horns and waving at us madly — so much for top secret. I thought of my father and how he must have felt sailing out of Sydney Harbour all those years ago. I remembered waving him off, holding onto Grandmother Polson with one hand and throwing streamers with the other. Finally it was my turn.

Onboard, conditions were splendid: we lived in cabins, slept in real beds and dined at tables boasting linen cloths and menus. It was like being a guest on a luxury hotel afloat. We reached Fremantle a week later, where O'Neill — who had arrived by train days ahead of us with an advance party — was waiting for us on the wharf. We greeted him with a mighty chorus of 'Peggy O'Neill', our regiment's unofficial anthem. A far cry from the grandeur of the *Katoomba*, we transferred to a Dutch troopship, the *Sibajak*. We had to adjust to sleeping in closely slung hammocks, our bodies sagging in rows above the same long mess benches where we ate our meals.

As we set sail from Fremantle, I remember hearing the mellow sound of a woman singing:

> *Now is the hour,*
> *When we must say goodbye.*
> *Soon you'll be sailing, far across the sea.*
> *While you're away,*

Oh please remember me,
When you return,
You'll find me waiting here . . . [4]

'Now is the Hour' was a favourite tune at social concerts, usually the last one played of an evening and always very emotional. We fell into a companionable silence, immersing ourselves in the words being carried across the water; her lonely voice becoming softer as we sailed further from the shore. Memories crowded our minds, reminding us of the many things we would miss of home.

There was little time to dwell on emotions though, we were flat out just doing our jobs and continuing our training. The officers had to develop a new regimental organisation for the 3-inch mortars: from the basics of determining the structure of a mortar regiment through to deployment, as well as detailing tactics and procedures, while the men had to undergo intensive training on the new weapons for which they would never hold any affection. They had to learn how to handle the mortars, assemble them, look after them and clean them. They also continued training on machine-guns, assembling and dismantling them while blindfolded to ensure they were prepared for night warfare.

Every morning I conducted sick parades, when any men who had become ill over night would report to me for assessment. The rest of my day usually involved tending to the sick, checking on Jim Armstrong and the RAP team, and conducting lectures on topics ranging from hygiene and first aid to the risk of acquiring sexually transmitted diseases from the fleshpots of Malaya (even though, officially, our destination remained undisclosed).

Blackout conditions were maintained onboard at all times to prevent us from being spotted by enemy submarines. Throughout the day, when the sun was burning high in the sky above us, we unbuttoned our khaki shirts and rolled up our sleeves while we worked. During recreation time men filed below deck to strip off their shirts, rest, read or play cards in a fog of cigarette smoke and sweat. We opened all the portholes to allow cool air to circulate. Once Fremantle had disappeared behind us, I felt for the first time the thrill of being officially, and finally, abroad. Captain C.R.B. Richards, NX70273, was on his way to war.

PART TWO

FROM SOLDIERS TO SLAVES

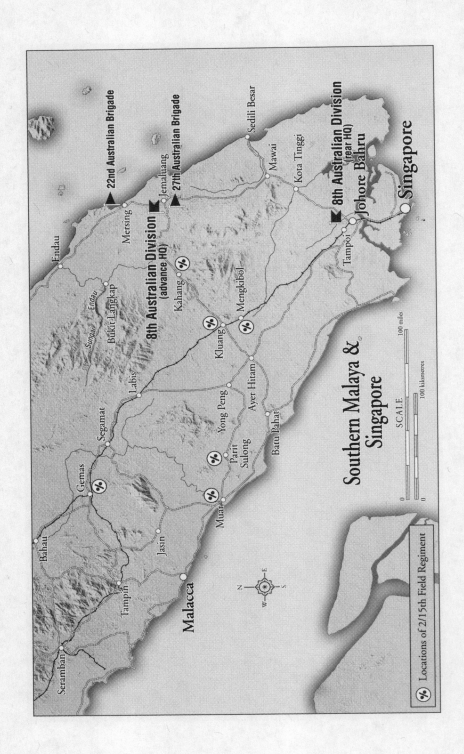

Southern Malaya & Singapore

22nd Australian Brigade

27th Australian Brigade

8th Australian Division (advance HQ)

8th Australian Division (rear HQ)

Singapore

Johore Bahru

Tampoi

Kota Tinggi

Mawai

Sedili Besar

Jemaluang

Mersing

Endau

Kahang

Mengkibol

Kluang

Yong Peng

Ayer Hitam

Parit Sulong

Batu Pahat

Muar

Bukit Langkap

Sungai Endau

Labis

Segamat

Gemas

Bahau

Jasin

Tampin

Seramban

Malacca

N
W — E
S

SCALE

0   100 miles

0   100 kilometres

% Locations of 2/15th Field Regiment

CHAPTER FOUR

THE MALAYAN CAMPAIGN
August 1941–February 1942

Locals laden with hessian sacks across their narrow shoulders passed us in the streets. Already accustomed to men in uniform flooding into their country, they were indifferent to our presence. I can still remember the smoky smell of unfamiliar spices as we watched men cooking kebabs over charcoal fires in the streets. The humidity was overwhelming, the heat equally so; our uniforms damp upon our backs with sweat. And then there was the rain: arriving every afternoon, out of the blue it seemed, belting down for about half an hour and then stopping as suddenly as it had started. Singapore was a strange place to those of us who had never before left home.

Upon arrival on 15 August, we had been greeted by the Deputy Assistant Director of Medical Services (DADMS), Lieutenant Colonel Glyn White, and officers from Division Headquarters before being transported to a tented camp in Nee Soon (in the grounds of a regular British artillery unit). Here we found the British officers relaxing in a palatial mess hall that featured highly polished cedar furniture, lounges, libraries and all sorts of other fancy trimmings, not to mention an ever-ready supply of native servants. We dubbed it 'Buckingham Palace' and wondered if the Brits needed reminding of where they were and why they were there.

The British officers evidently believed they were entitled to significant special privileges over their troops — their mess hall being the first of many examples we would witness. I can only speculate that the history of the British Army played some part. During the eighteenth century, British soldiers were recruited from the poorest members of society, including criminals, while officers were usually drawn from the echelons of the gentry and were allowed to 'purchase' their commissions. Frequently units were formed by a squire and his farmers. From what we could see, the old class system was still very much at play. Their way was not the Australian way. In the British tradition, the relationship between an officer and his men was one of master–servant, but in the Australian Army it was more one of master–friend. As an officer, you were considered the boss, but outside of working hours, friendships could be egalitarian. The British officers, as a class all on their own, became immediately 'offside' with us.

In Nee Soon I maintained my commitment to first-aid training and hygiene discipline. I ordered the men to continue sterilising their dixies and eating irons in boiling water before and after meals; to wear their sleeves rolled down to prevent mosquito bites; to clear rubbish and get rid of any stagnant water to prevent flies and mosquitoes from breeding. Thanks to the information imparted to us by Reg Nutt and Jim McNiven before departing Australia, we purchased tins of Johnson's Baby Powder, neck towels and wooden clogs for every man (courtesy of the Comforts Fund) to help prevent tinea and other skin problems. It was soon considered almost criminal for any man to be found barefoot anywhere except in bed. Little by little the men were coming to understand the importance of such procedures.

The same couldn't be said of our British counterparts. Not long after we arrived, one of the British medical officers mentioned to me that he was having a problem with flies in one of the kitchens on an isolated anti-aircraft position on the island. He believed the source of the problem was the Sultan's stables (located a good eight kilometres away!). I offered to take a look at the kitchen in question and the medical officer led the way.

I looked inside the rubbish bin and then the sink. 'Where does the sink drain?' I asked.

The medical officer shrugged. 'I don't know.' I invited him to follow me outside, which he did, albeit reluctantly. The effluent from the sink was allowed to flow straight out into the open ground. I picked up a stick and poked at some of the maggots. 'These will be flies any time soon,' I said. It was obvious these Brits had been living and training in only concrete barracks for quite some time and that they were unprepared for living in isolated positions. My opinion of the British officers continued to head south.

In early September, after nearly a month of becoming acclimatised to the humid heat of the tropics, leeches, daily rainfall, and ongoing training with the mortars, we were sent to Tampin in southern Malaya, situated at the junction of northern Johore and the State of Malacca. Here our jungle training began in earnest, including live shoots. I made periodic visits to the 10th Australian General Hospital (10 AGH) in nearby Malacca to attend compulsory conferences and seminars. Resentment between RMOs and those we called 'doctors in uniform' quickly emerged. We did not appreciate being given advice, especially from the junior specialists who were working in a hospital environment — behaving, it seemed to us, as if they were at the Royal Prince Alfred Hospital back home — while we were out in the *jungle*. We thought they had as much to learn from us as we did from them.

ALL SOULS' DAY, 2 November 1941, will forever remain a day I will regret for the rest of my life. It started well. Despite mounting concern about when Japan might pounce on Singapore, we still had the luxury of occasional rest and relaxation days. Des and I were on leave so decided to take a day trip, like tourists, to nearby Segamat. Nearly every town in Malaya seemed to have a little club where the plantation owners and managers used to gather for food and grog, and Des and I enjoyed a relaxing day at the club in Segamat, eating well and catching up as friends, off-duty.

We drove back to camp that evening and as soon as Des and I walked into the mess we knew something was wrong; it was buzzing with conversation and the faces of our men were blank. A fellow officer delivered the news: John O'Neill, our beloved and well-respected commanding officer, was dead. The details followed in a string of facts: O'Neill was driving to a social event in a nearby town that morning. He lost control of his vehicle on a corner of a dirt road. The vehicle rolled. He died shortly afterwards at the 10 AGH. There were three other officers with him in the car, none of whom was seriously hurt.

Aside from grief, the most powerful emotion I felt was guilt. There was a very strict rule, even before we left Australia: under no circumstances was an officer to drive a vehicle, except with the express permission of the CO. At home, O'Neill had allowed me to drive his private car when I was visiting nurses in the nearby medical unit, and in Malaya, on our days off, I used to drive his car for him when we were on social visits. He was very conscious of the fact that, as RMO, I considered myself 'on duty' 24 hours a day seven days a week. If we attended a dinner or a club, he knew I would sit on a scotch with a water chaser. I was the safest driver on whom he could always rely. He should never have been driving his own vehicle. Over and over in my mind ran the thought, 'If only I had been there to drive him.' I was overwhelmed with regret.

O'Neill was laid to rest the following day in Malacca after a full regimental military funeral service at the Saint Francis Xavier Church. Following his casket, we slow-marched from the church to the cemetery. Slow marching is no easy task — the tempo of each man needs to be perfect while you struggle to balance on one foot at a time — and it seemed to take forever to reach the graveside, where Padre Brendan Rogers conducted a final service. It rained like stink: we were all saturated.

I cannot recall how we conducted the wake, or what we said to comfort one another. Memory is a strange thing; there are so many details about this day and the mourning that followed which I just cannot remember. My mind has somehow blocked out the memories which are too painful to accept. I'm sure a psychiatrist could explain this, but I certainly can't. This reaction was true not only for me, but of nearly all our regiment. Years ago when we were writing our regimental history, I asked many of our men what happened on the day of the accident and at the funeral which followed. No one had a clear recollection.

Much-needed good news arrived the following week with the announcement that Major John Wright, our second in command (2 i/c), had been promoted to lieutenant colonel and was to be our new commanding officer, and John Workman — a vibrant and fearless personality — was promoted to 2 i/c. Wright had served in the First World War initially as a light horseman and later in the Flying Corps as a fighter pilot. Known as 'Gentleman John', as 2 i/c he had been the perfect foil to the larrikin O'Neill. In turn, Workman, who was every bit the character O'Neill had been, became the perfect complement to Wright. It was a relief to have two such men as leaders following our shattering loss. Further good news arrived later in the month when we learned we would be receiving British-made 25-pounder gun-howitzers. These gun-howitzers were both modern and, most importantly, the artillery on which the men had been originally trained to work.

RUMOURS THAT 'THE JAPS are coming' had been flying for some time by now. We knew the Imperial Japanese Army (IJA) was close, but we didn't know just how soon they would attack. A reckless mix of propaganda and tall tales about our enemy had resulted in much discussion since leaving Australia. Word spread that these 'little yellow men' suffered from night blindness, that their guns only fired small bullets and that they couldn't shoot straight. Most of us were aware of Japan's military aggression in China — in particular the rape of the Nationalist Chinese capital, Nanking — so few genuinely believed the circulating party-lines, but all of us would soon be disillusioned by the strength and determination of our adversaries.

During the day on 29 November our regiment received the code word 'Awake' via our sigs (signallers), which meant that the international situation had deteriorated and we needed to be ready to move into battle stations at six hours' notice. Later in the day the code word 'Armour' was received, signalling that war with Japan was imminent. The Malayan campaign was about to begin for real.

I was not fearful of impending action. There is no question I was nervous — action would be new to all of us, aside from the handful of veterans from the First World War — but I accepted the arrival of our enemy as inevitable. Indoctrinated in military procedures, I was determined to do my job. It might sound implausible, not being scared of losing your life, but that is the way I remember it. At that time fear was still secondary to taking care of my men and obeying orders. Countless journalists since have questioned me over the matter. 'You must all have been so frightened,' they say. 'Have you ever been to war?' I ask them. 'It wasn't the way you think it was.' At this stage, moving into battle stations, we were yet to come face to face with our enemy; there would be plenty of time ahead to be afraid.

Days passed, all of us in a controlled state of anxiety. No man voiced unease about heading into action; it would have been seen as a sign of weakness, the breaking of an unspoken code. We were expected to be soldiers, first and foremost, and we didn't want to let our mates down. We knew things were hotting up when the men of our regiment who acted as sentries, keeping watch over a limited area of our camp (but without live ammunition), were replaced by security guards. Our guards worked in pairs, armed with rifles, fixed bayonets, and live ammunition, patrolling vast areas at irregular intervals, looking for any signs of our enemy. I remember one of our overly enthusiastic guards firing the first bullet, his partner on duty quickly following suit. The sound of the shots ringing out throughout the silent countryside was enough to bring all of us to our feet before it was quickly declared a false alarm. The guards in question swore they saw movement in the scrub before letting their bullets fly. But it wasn't the Japanese, more than likely the wag of a stray dog, or just active young imaginations responding to the increasing pressure.

By the afternoon of 5 December, our regiment received the code word 'Seaview', indicating that a declaration of war was expected hourly; we were to be prepared to move at a half hour's notice. Action was another step closer, but what we were most concerned about was that not all of the associated gun stores for the 25-pounders had arrived: it seemed our guns would not be ready in time. At 1700 hours on 6 December we received the code word 'Raffles', which meant 'Go' — but still we had to await orders. There was no scramble. War, we were learning, could take quite some time.

The following day I made my first diary entry in a small loose-leaf notebook.[1] There was little time to record much detail; I logged the code signals we had received since 'Awake' and then quickly tucked the diary into my pack for safekeeping. We received our movement orders later that same day and by midnight we were on our way to battle stations, armed with the much-maligned 3-inch mortars as well as our 25-pounder gun-howitzers — which would remain useless until we obtained the necessary supplies.

Two troops from our regiment were sent along the east coast (about 250 kilometres away) while the rest of us kept to the main road. We travelled bumper-to-bumper in motor convoy, more than 100 vehicles slowly snaking their way through the night. Drivers frequently had to prod sergeants in the front seat beside them every time they nodded off. Men took turns at sleeping. The journey through unfamiliar terrain was made even more difficult by sloping rain and the need to maintain blackout conditions. It was difficult to see in front of our own vehicle and we had to be careful not to bump into those ahead. Our destination was Mengkibol Estate, a rubber plantation near Kluang, which we reached just as the sun was rising. My boots sank into the claggy ground when I climbed out of our truck; black mud was thickly slapped to its tyres. Evergreen rubber trees enclosed us, their narrow trunks sprouting skywards in widely planted rows; there were corridors of boggy slush in between.

John Wright soon received orders that our regiment was to be further dispersed. All of a sudden our war was moving quickly. Troops were sent from Mengkibol Estate to defend aerodromes at Kluang and nearby Kahang, with other troops in reserve near Kluang, and Advance Regimental Headquarters was sent to Jemaluang, north-east of Kluang. Rear Regimental Headquarters was to remain at Mengkibol. Just as O'Neill and I had anticipated before leaving Australia, our regiment was now widely scattered — covering a front of more than 250 kilometres. Our extensive first-aid training of battery and troop medical orderlies had been vindicated.

On the morning of 8 December, all of us sleep deprived from constant movement orders, we learned of Japan's devastating attack on the US naval base of Pearl Harbor. We couldn't believe the news. It was a mystery to us how Pearl Harbor could have been caught napping when we had received a week's worth of code signals. It was now, it seemed, truly a *world* war.

THE JAPANESE INVASION OF Malaya began on 8 December with the landing of troops in Kota Bharu in the north, followed by the arrival of more troops in Patani and Singora in Siam (Thailand). British and Indian troops copped the worst of the initial onslaught, as the three Japanese divisions — the Imperial Guards Division, and the 5th and 18th Japanese Divisions — moved south in three prongs. The Imperial Guards Division moved down the west coast, both by land and sea; the 18th Division moved down the east coast by land and sea, while the 5th Division moved generally down the centre of the Malayan peninsula.

The general Japanese tactic was to attack, with mostly unopposed air and tank support, and when any resistance was encountered, to outflank the defenders with the object of cutting them off, encircling and then annihilating them. Often the outflanking movements were conducted through dense jungle — previously believed by Allied forces to be impenetrable — utilising tracks and the assistance of a well-organised fifth column of Chinese and Malays sympathetic to the Japanese.

While the Japanese forced their way down towards Singapore, the 8th Division AIF — to which our regiment belonged — commanded by Lieutenant General Gordon Bennett, remained in southern Malaya. Bennett, a former Militia man who had proven his worth in the First World War, only had two of his three brigades and their supporting units in Malaya because the third had been split up, posted among Ambon, Rabaul, Timor and Darwin. Bennett would never have control over a complete division.

While fighting raged to our north, we lay in waiting, our men in place but without a definite role to play as yet. Jumpy guards continued to fire pot shots into the bush at night when they heard movements. We couldn't see our enemy, but we knew they were on their way. Outside of our own Anglo-Saxon comfort zone, we struggled to differentiate between the Japanese and other Asian men in Malaya. The IJA could easily infiltrate our locations without us being any the wiser.

With Christmas fast approaching, Wright charged me with an important mission: cashed-up with a roll of Singapore Straits Settlement dollars (again thanks to the Comforts Fund), I was ordered to buy goodies with the aim of boosting the morale of sleepless troops. I drove a truck to Singapore and loaded plum puddings and beer into the back. It was an important moment in the history of our regiment: for many of our men it would be their last Christmas. Because the puddings and beer were purchased by the Comforts Fund, the men viewed their gifts as a link with home and the small treats ensured a true sense of Christmas cheer pervaded. The best present of all, though, arrived with the order that our men were to switch back to the versatile 25-pounders: the missing gun supplies had been trickling in over the past couple of weeks, and now, at last, it was time to calibrate the fair-dinkum artillery.

DURING THE REST OF December and early January, we continued to await our enemy. The men became increasingly proficient with the 25-pounders, and, in the process, our regiment was converted from two batteries (each with three troops) to three batteries (each of two troops) to conform to the British military establishment for field artillery. Our 29th and 30th Batteries moved into the Gemas area in central Johore, while the newly formed 65th Battery was detached to the west coast, under the command of the 45th Indian Brigade.

The 2/15th did not fight as an 'intact regiment'. As a result, I didn't function in the ordinary role of an RMO: my job was a roving commission. Luckily for me, when new vehicles had arrived in early January, I managed to 'acquire' one simply by offering to drive it. With the war officially *on*, I no longer sought permission to drive a vehicle and no one tried to stop me. I drove my truck, stocked with the ten tea chests of medical supplies I had shipped over from Australia, between our widely dispersed men, maintaining communications with the troop and battery medical orderlies. Communications by wireless were very unreliable, especially in hilly jungle; only local field telephones were operational. I was responsible for personally advising the medical orderlies of the ever-changing locations of the medical units and battalion RAPs in their vicinity. I was also offering medical advice and replenishing their medical supplies. I was not yet seeing any casualties or illnesses: if any of the men became unwell they were evacuated to the nearest field ambulance or casualty clearing station.

I spent each night at the RAP with Jim Armstrong and headed off to Brigade Headquarters first thing every morning to find out 'where the war was at', so to speak. Every day the enemy was getting closer, heading towards Singapore, and our units of men were constantly on the move. During the day I was mostly on my own, driving through the jungle with a map to guide me — my mapping experience, thanks to my father and the Artillery Survey Company, was a great help. The roads through the jungle were mainly sealed with deep ditches on either side. Driving along without the protection of a canopy, I felt exposed: forever expecting a Japanese soldier to spring out of a ditch, or a sniper to take a shot from the safety of the forest. I couldn't see the enemy, but I could feel them hiding somewhere amongst those handsome trees. Every journey was a mental obstacle course and all I could do was keep driving, the incentive always being to get to my men.

At no time did I wear a Red Cross patch, nor would I display the symbol on my truck or on the RAP vehicle. We had heard reports that the Japanese were treating the symbol as a 'bullseye' target for attacks. Our RAP was usually adjacent to either the Advance Headquarters or the Rear Headquarters. We knew the Japanese could track Red Cross vehicles through the jungle, identify where they stopped and then bomb or shell the area, hoping they might wipe out our headquarters.

On 14 January, our 30th Battery, along with the 2/30th Battalion, was involved in the Gemas ambush: the first time the AIF would meet the Japanese in action in Malaya. Late in the afternoon, while Australian troops lay in waiting, approximately a thousand unsuspecting bicycle-riding Japanese fell into a carefully planned trap west of the village of Gemas. After the first few hundred Japanese had crossed a wooden bridge over the Gemencheh River, the Australians blew the bridge and then unleashed hand grenades and machine-gun fire on the surprised Japanese, who had nowhere to run.[2] The Gemas battle was considered an outstanding military success by the infantry, with an estimated 600 Japanese killed. For the field artillery, it was a disaster: we lost three out of our four 25-pounders when they became irretrievably bogged after solid rainfall.[3] My friend Des Makepeace, by then a battery captain, was cut off for three days at Gemas. He caught a spent Japanese bullet in his mouth and was lucky to suffer only chipped teeth.

On the morning of the Gemas ambush, I paid a routine visit to Muar, on the west coast, to check on Corporal F.J. 'Pinkey' Rhodes, one of my medical orderlies, and to top up his medical supplies. I was accompanied by Sergeant Mick Petchell (aka 'Shivery Mick'), our pay sergeant, whom I had persuaded to come along for the ride. By this time, I was accustomed to looking ahead *and* above when travelling along open roads, always on the watch for the metallic glint of enemy aircraft overhead. During our return trip to headquarters, on the Bakri–Parit Sulong causeway, we saw Japanese fighters swooping down towards us. In quick succession bullets spattered down the road ahead. The Japanese had been an invisible enemy to me up until this moment, but now the goggled faces of those fighter pilots seemed to be looking straight at us. We pulled over and dived into the ditches beside the road for protection, our hearts thumping. It was my first close call.

THE 'TRIUMPH' OF THE Gemas ambush immediately resulted in increased Japanese pressure on Muar, where our 65th Battery remained under the command of the 45th Indian Brigade. The 2/29th Battalion was sent to assist them. The Allied men at Muar were given orders to hold up the Japanese for one week to enable the main body of withdrawing British and Indian forces to avoid encirclement on their way south. They were reinforced by more Allied troops the following day.[4] The Muar battle well and truly unfolded during the ensuing week. I soon realised that the strafing Shivery Mick and I had experienced was a prelude to the mass assault by the Japanese Imperial Guards Division that followed the next day.

By the end of the week, the battle was moving towards a tragic conclusion at Parit Sulong, south-east of Muar. By this time, I had received word that our 65th Battery, together with a beleaguered column of men led by Lieutenant Colonel Charles Anderson,[5] was in trouble — their whereabouts were unknown. Since our last close call, Shivery Mick had made himself unavailable any time I requested a driving companion, so I invited Lieutenant Russ Ewin, our sigs officer, to accompany me on a road trip to see if we could help find our missing men.

As we approached Parit Sulong, Russ and I came across the 2nd Loyals Battalion (a regular British garrison unit stationed in Singapore), which was reportedly preparing to launch a counterattack against the Japanese Imperial Guards Division. I can still picture them lolling about, their bodies relaxed beneath the shade of rubber trees. Initially, Russ and I were in awe. We thought it was marvellous they could be so cool before launching a counterattack. We called out from the truck to a couple of the officers, asking if they knew the location of our missing men. They shook their heads. I can't remember what they said, it was their tone of voice I will never forget: utter apathy. At that moment we realised they weren't cool, just uninterested, even ill prepared. These were the most advanced of our troops and they were seemingly careless. Cold anger rushed through me. Incensed, Russ and I decided to keep driving into the unknown.

The jungle is a pretty quiet place: you don't hear the calls of wildlife like you do in the Australian bush. On this day, the silence was deathly. The sound of our engine was painfully loud against the hushed backdrop. Neither of us was willing to admit that we were starting to feel frightened: we knew we were now well forward of our own troops and possibly in Japanese territory. We drove on a little further still, looking straight ahead; the silence continued. There was no sign of our men. After a few more minutes, without speaking to Russ, I turned the truck around and we headed back. It is hard to convey the way we felt. Even now the whole excursion feels like a delusion; the details have vanished. We were sitting ducks, both Russ and I knew that, and we had been very foolish to keep driving. We were just so angry that nothing was being done to find and assist our withdrawing troops. It was certainly not our objective to take on the Japanese Imperial Guards Division single-handed!

We later learned we had been almost certainly within sight and range of the large force of Japanese that was holding the high ground on a defile on the east bank of the Simpang Kiri River, as well as the Parit Sulong Bridge (our enemy had moved ahead of the withdrawing Allies — down the coast and then inland). Why they held their fire, I will never know. Rumours had been swirling amongst our men that the Japanese were sending decoy trucks into Allied territory to draw fire in order to reveal their enemy's position. Perhaps they thought we were doing the same thing. It was my second lucky escape.

We soon discovered that the 45th Indian Brigade and its supporting units had been rapidly overcome by the Imperial Guards Division. And, as history records, Anderson's stranded column had no choice but to break up and make its own way through the jungle to AIF lines, with the order: 'Every man for himself.' During the battle of Muar, our regiment lost 39 men from the 65th Battery (including its commander, Major Bill Julius), and close to 640 Allied men from the rest of Anderson's besieged column were also lost.[6] All were killed in action or missing believed killed in action.

The tragic cost of the battle of Muar had not been in vain: the men had succeeded in holding up the Japanese for nearly a week, enabling retreating British and Indian troops to escape almost certain annihilation. The Japanese sustained heavy losses in the process and, in retaliation, massacred approximately 110 Australians and 40 Indians at Parit Sulong in one of the worst of the many atrocities inflicted by the Japanese during the Second World War.[7] The remnants of the AIF made their way to Yong Peng and then to Singapore. Some were captured by the Japanese and sent to Pudu Prison in Kuala Lumpur; others were later listed as missing believed killed in action.

During the last week of January, our regiment supported the 27th Brigade in a fighting withdrawal to Singapore Island. It was not unusual to move at least once every night, sometimes even two or three times: we became accustomed to living on bugger-all sleep. Regardless of the overwhelming strength of the Japanese, the men remained determined: 'We're better than those bastards.'

The last of our regiment, led by CO Lieutenant Colonel John Wright, crossed the causeway from Johore to Singapore Island on the night of 31 January/1 February to find that the defence of the supposedly 'impregnable' island was a myth. No defensive barbed wire had been laid nor had any defensive trenches been dug in preparation for us.

After an unrelenting artillery barrage covering the north-west segment of the island — described by some First World War veterans as the heaviest they had ever experienced — the Japanese landed on the island in large numbers on 8 February. Tanks followed soon after. The onslaught was catastrophic. Sixteen Japanese battalions, with five in reserve, were faced by just two AIF battalions with only one in reserve over a front of ten kilometres. The overwhelming number of Japanese, their unopposed air attacks and their tank support made the defenders' task a mission impossible.

On 11 February I was visiting our sick and wounded in the 10 AGH and 13 AGH when I received word that Jim McNiven, the doctor I had met in Sydney prior to embarkation, was at the Goodward Park Hotel. Eager to catch up with him, I made my way to the colonial-style hotel dressed in full battle gear — complete with tin hat, and revolver and hand grenades attached to my belt. I found Jim in the lounge area: he and his male guests were dressed in tuxedos, their lady companions in glamorous dinner gowns, standing at the bar playing liar dice (a gambling game). Here they were, partying in majestic surroundings, knocking back drinks and backslapping while their countrymen were losing their lives. Didn't they realise there was a war going on, that Singapore was under siege? If I wasn't so stunned I might have laughed.

Jim greeted me warmly, 'Richards! Have a drink, old chap. Tell me what you're drinking?' The dice-players seemed oblivious to my attire; perhaps they were maintaining the British stiff upper lip, or were simply in denial. Whatever it was, their lack of concern made me feel like a bull in a china shop. Speechless, I waved and left them to it. I returned to our Regimental Headquarters to discover it had been bombed during the day. All that was left was a heap of rubble and ruin. It was like waking up to reality after a strange dream. There had been some injuries, but patients were evacuated by the time I arrived. Anticipating the attack, many of our men had taken cover in the slit trenches nearby, escaping death. This was the first attack we had experienced on our headquarters — and yet another blaring signal that the war was not going our way.

FRIDAY, 13 FEBRUARY WAS a very black Friday, with 27 Japanese bombers arriving in formations, dubbed the 'Singapore Express', causing incredible damage to the city and its civilian population. When dawn broke the following day, the situation worsened, with still more concentrated bombing. Everyone had gone to ground. We hadn't had enough time to dig any slit trenches before the attacks so I was under the base of a large tree with Teddy Edwards, a dispatch rider, on one side and Vic Carter, the RAP driver, on the other. We lay there listening to the bombs: they were incessant and bloody loud. When we started to hear *whooooshing* followed by a high-pitched scream and then a long whistling sound, we knew they were getting too close. We kept as low to the ground as possible, hoping that the storm would soon pass.

Now I was afraid — in action, everyone is afraid, to say you weren't would be nonsense, but I knew I couldn't allow the fear to paralyse me or affect my judgment. Ted, Vic and I called out to one another from time to time. No more than, 'You okay?' but it was reassuring to get a response. Sweat ran all over our bodies as the bombs slammed down around us, pocking the earth. The smell of dust and TNT hung in the air. I didn't think the bombs could get any closer — but within moments they were. I felt a stream of wind brush my scalp followed by the sound of metal fragments peppering into the tree above me. Then Teddy let out a loud gasp but I couldn't afford a glance: I needed to keep my face planted firmly in the dirt.

When the planes finally passed, I lifted my head tentatively. Bomb fragments were lodged in the trunk of my tree; they had missed my head by millimetres. Teddy was kneeling beside me, his calf shredded by a fragment, while Vic had received one through his mess tin, which was clipped to his belt. (Vic, a true believer, carried his Bible inside his tin and, remarkably, the shell fragment had become lodged in the Bible. Someone was looking after him, it seemed.) Not so lucky was another one of our blokes nearby, who was killed during the bombing. At the time, it was the worst casualty I had seen: few things in life are as ugly as a violent death. We lost several men that day and our CO Lieutenant Colonel John Wright was blown through the door of a bombproof shelter at Regimental Headquarters on Tanglin Hill; he was lucky to only suffer a lacerated knee. Another dispatch rider was sent to find me and take me back to Regimental Headquarters to stitch Wright's knee. I sat on the back of the motorcycle, gripping on for dear life while we sped along roads scarred with craters.

The Japanese now controlled the reservoirs, denying Allied forces access to water, and our ammunition and food supplies were running low. With no more land to which to withdraw, we realised there was no possibility of evacuation. There was rarely a lull in Japanese bombing and shelling and the civilian population had next to no chance of escape as their city was hammered from the sky. Singapore was falling but we continued to fight. Some of the less experienced soldiers were writing letters to loved ones and saying prayers. One of the many things I recall during our final hours of fighting was the reaction of some of the new recruits who had arrived in Singapore only days before the end. Some were so raw they didn't even know how to load a rifle properly. I can still picture one poor lad; he'd gone bonkers — that was what we called it at the time — as a result of shell shock. He tried to claw his way bare-handed through a bitumen road.

ON SUNDAY, 15 FEBRUARY, the fatal and final day, artillery fire ceased at 1130 hours but the bombing continued. All the AIF were ordered to Tanglin Barracks and the Artillery assembled on the golf links nearby. Meanwhile, I arrived at 8th Division Headquarters in the early evening to report to the Assistant Director of Medical Services (ADMS), Colonel Alfred Derham. A veteran of the First World War, 'Daddy' Derham was a kind man who was very supportive of his RMOs. I waited outside while a guard announced my arrival.

Before long, I was watching the staff car of the GOC (general officer commanding) screaming towards Headquarters, then jolt to a stop in front of me. Lieutenant General Gordon Bennett, accompanied by Major Charles Moses and other staff officers, rushed past me into Division Headquarters. Left to wait outside, I could hear the scraping of boots on floorboards, voices murmuring, and what sounded like coins being dropped into a metal dish (in fact it was the sound of ammunition being emptied from their revolvers into a tin bucket). I couldn't make out what they were saying, but I assumed orders were being issued for surrender. While none of us wanted to give up, I think every Allied man knew our campaign was finished. We'd been beaten and beaten badly.

After about half an hour, the door opened and Bennett and his team again hurried past me. They were farewelled by the senior officers who remained, including Derham and Boots Callaghan. They all looked grim. Boots didn't see me; Derham did. Boots headed back inside and Derham walked over to personally tell me the news that the British General Arthur Percival had surrendered unconditionally to the Japanese commander General Tomoyuki Yamashita. Singapore had officially fallen: the Malayan campaign was over. He also informed me that the GOC had just relinquished command to Brigadier Callaghan (soon to be Major General). Bennett was going to attempt an escape to Australia to advise of the details of the campaign.

'This is the beginning of God knows what, Richards,' Derham said. He spoke highly and warmly of his medical officers, nurses and medical orderlies; then he put his left hand on my shoulder and shook my hand.

'Rowley,' he said, 'I know of your work with the regiment. I thank you.'

I saluted, and with difficulty said, 'Good night, sir.' I about-turned rapidly to hide my tears.

CHAPTER FIVE

INTO CAPTIVITY
Changi
February–May 1942

Back at Regimental Headquarters on Tanglin golf links, John Wright returned from Division Headquarters that evening and called a conference of all officers to announce the details of the unconditional surrender. Following orders from Lieutenant General Gordon Bennett, he instructed us to remain with our troops. 'There is to be no organised evacuation or attempt to escape,' he said. 'If caught, the Japanese penalty will be death.'

The consequences of capitulation started to pierce our numbed minds.

I made my way to the RAP to formally pass on the news to Jim Armstrong and the other orderlies. Their reaction was initially shock, quickly followed by relief — relief that the constant withdrawals had ended and relief that the massacre of civilians was over (or, at least, so we thought at the time). The Japanese now ruled Malaya and we were defeated men: prisoners of war with no clue as to what our fate might be. We had been ordered to surrender, and of course had no say in the matter, but it didn't stop many of us from feeling guilty, even humiliated — we knew we had failed. No army wants to be trounced by its enemy. We wandered around aimlessly, mostly in silence.

Later that same evening, Sergeant Wally Brown, the quartermaster sergeant and a recipient of the Victoria Cross in the First World War, approached Wright and all the officers at Regimental Headquarters.

'Thanks for the honour of serving with you. There's no way I'm going to become a prisoner of war for those little yellow bastards. I'm well armed,' he said, pointing to his machine gun, revolver and hand grenades, 'and will *never* be taken alive.' Wally, noise deaf as a result of the First World War, was quiet and unassuming; he was regarded as a role model by younger soldiers. Determined to serve his country for a second time, he was 54 years old when he enlisted in the Second AIF but had given his age as forty. We pleaded with him and his group of followers to change their minds, even attempting to restrain them physically, but for Wally and his men, there was no turning back. They walked off into the darkness.[1]

Exhaustion finally overcame us. We had been in action continuously for only four weeks but we had had very little sleep, or even rest: everyone was shattered. The adrenalin which had helped keep us awake for so long drained away and our disillusionment was temporarily suspended for sleep. I climbed into the passenger seat of my truck, put my head back on the seat and fell into a deep slumber.

THE FOLLOWING MORNING I woke to a world of unreality: I felt as though I had the mother of all hangovers — one which would last for days — and my ears were ringing. A 25-pounder rattling off 100 rounds of ammunition, one after the other, makes an awful lot of noise. The hammering of artillery is quite literally deafening, and being so close to gunfire damaged nearly all gunners, desensitising our hearing and causing a lifetime of tinnitus. The bombing had stopped, but sounds continued to buzz inside our ears.

Climbing out of my truck, my immediate thoughts turned to my job. I was lucky being a doctor as I still had specific responsibilities: my men still needed me in exactly the same role I had been trained to perform. Aside from commanding officers, medical officers and padres, all other men had been effectively made 'redundant' overnight. Many were wounded and a number were already suffering from malaria. All were experiencing mixed emotions: exhaustion, relief, disbelief, remorse at having surrendered but, perhaps surprisingly, not yet despair. While I was treating the sick, others spent the day attempting to obstruct our enemy: removing vital parts from our guns, putting sand and sugar in the petrol tanks and oil sumps of vehicles, and performing every other form of bastardy and sabotage they could think of to deny our equipment being of use to the Japanese. I dumped my revolver and hand grenades down a well. The rest of the day I spent in a daze.

The next day, we watched one of the British units passing by. There were numerous trucks bulging with officers' mess equipment: cane chairs, typewriters and no doubt a full set of cut glass, silver candlesticks, china and cutlery. Soon after, Lieutenant Theo Walker, the intelligence officer, brought instructions from Division Headquarters that we were to leave for Changi, some 25 kilometres away, at 1530 hours. Furthermore, *all* food and medical supplies were to be left behind, to be transported at a later date; no vehicles other than water carts were to be taken; and each man was only to bring whatever personal belongings he could carry on his own back during the long march ahead.

Wright, fuming over the blatant arrogance of the Brits, turned to Theo and said: 'I did not hear that order.' If it was okay for the Brits to take with them everything but the kitchen sink, then it was good enough for us, too. We left for Changi with four quartermaster trucks, a van loaded with food and three full water carts. I drove another truck crammed full of medical supplies. Gear of all sorts was piled high on top of all vehicles. I displayed the Red Cross on my truck for the first time: I thought it would help reinforce my status as RMO and at the very least couldn't now do any harm. If I was caught driving the contraband vehicle, at least I would have rank on my side; without rank, many of us assumed we would just be another nonentity to the Japanese.

The Japanese troops — who, like us, only days ago had been soldiers in combat — weren't particularly enthusiastic about their new responsibilities as sentinels. Some lined the road on the way to Changi, but there was no interaction between 'us and them', aside from a bit of harmless jeering on their behalf. Wright marched the entire 25 kilometres at the head of our regiment, leading his men, despite his wounded knee, while the CO of the 2/10th Field Regiment, Lieutenant Colonel Alfred 'Alf' Walsh, just out of hospital, rode with me. He chose to 'receive' instructions from Division Headquarters — to take only the permitted number of water carts and supplies — but was nevertheless happy to ride in my illicit vehicle!

The British had been ordered to move into a designated compound at Changi Gaol, while the Australians were to move into Selarang Barracks and other satellite camps within the Changi area. Our regiment was bound for Birdwood Camp, located a short distance from both the gaol and Selarang Barracks. I had been issued with a detailed route map, but in the event it was really just a case of follow-the-leader. With a total of approximately 85,000 prisoners of war to be detained — including approximately 17,000 men of the 8th Division AIF — we journeyed at a snail's pace.[2]

We arrived at the entrance gates of Birdwood Camp in the early hours of 18 February. It was dark, the headlights of our vehicles the only relief against the black sky. Our regiment was met by staff officers from Division Headquarters (which was located in the nearby Selarang area). Upon sighting our vehicles loaded with supplies, they were incensed. Wright was upbraided in front of his column of men. I couldn't see what was happening, but many of the men could hear and word quickly spread down our line about the dressing down our CO received. It was not so much what was said to Wright but the fact that a junior major was criticising a commanding officer in front of his own men. True to his name, Gentleman John did not retaliate. He spoke quietly and convincingly and another staff officer relented, allowing our vehicles through on the condition that all rations and medical supplies be handed over to Division Headquarters later that morning. Wright provided us with a lesson in the importance of maintaining self-control in the face of adversity — a skill all of us would need to refine if we were to survive imprisonment by the IJA.

BIRDWOOD CAMP WAS A shambles: the area had obviously been attacked from the air and most of the bamboo huts had been damaged. With hundreds of men milling about in such a confined space, our area resembled an Oriental bazaar. We were still mentally stunned — and felt powerless — but thanks to the leadership of Wright we soon recognised the need to keep our minds busy if we had any chance of restoring morale. Officers ordered men to focus on 'housekeeping': tidying up the camp, repairing holes in the *attap* (dried palm leaves thatched together) walls and roofs of our huts, and digging boreholes or slit trenches to serve as latrines. Our 2 i/c, John Workman, assembled a squad of men to rebuild one of the damaged huts. In the aftermath of the bombing there was no shortage of scrap material lying about which they could use. Workman and his team built a dummy bamboo and *attap* wall inside the hut, creating a sizeable cavity in the process. Inside, a considerable quantity of rations and some medical supplies were cached to foil not only the Japanese but also Division Headquarters. Another wall was then built to conceal the store. Workman, always one to seize an opportunity, wasn't going to allow Division Headquarters to knock off our treasured supplies.

Later in the morning, true to their word, staff officers from Division Headquarters confiscated the remainder of the rations and medical supplies that were still in our trucks, including masses of Atebrin, a valuable drug used for the prevention and treatment of malaria. The staff officers organised their own working party to bury the supplies to ensure that the Japanese wouldn't find them. Livid over the loss of our medical supplies, a select few of our men took it upon themselves to secretly follow the staff officers to find out where the stash was being buried.

At Changi, our Japanese keepers remained, for the most part, absent. They used our existing ranks and AIF command structures for their own means. They issued orders to our Division Headquarters, which in turn handed down orders to their own officers. Division Headquarters was the meat in the sandwich. Being emissaries for the Japanese, they had the unenviable task of forever being the bearers of bad news to their own men, but following their chastising of our own CO we could feel no sympathy for them.

ONE OF THE FIRST things we did at Changi was account for our men. A regimental roll book had been commenced when the regiment was first formed and, since then, a total of 828 names had been recorded. By the time of surrender, only 674 were present in Birdwood Camp. It was difficult to come to terms with the loss of so many lives: nineteen had been killed in action; twelve were missing believed killed; 99 were missing; two had been accidentally killed; four had died from wounds; and eighteen had been repatriated to Australia.[3]

So many of our mates had become ugly statistics in a bitter campaign, but we could not afford to dwell on our losses. No man was immune to sadness, but in the years to come we would learn to accept death on a daily basis as inevitable. Establishing a routine helped me maintain my own sense of purpose. I conducted sick parades every morning, immediately after reveille. Any man who had become ill overnight reported to his local sergeant, who would then fill in the appropriate form (Army Form A46) and order the sick man to go on parade at our Regimental Headquarters, where we had established our RAP inside a small hut. Each fellow waited on parade for his name to be called before he could come into the RAP to explain his problem. Jim Armstrong, my sergeant, was always by my side. As I examined each man, I instructed Jim as to the appropriate treatment — in these early days it was most often iodine, a couple of aspirin or a bandage, and then we sent the man on his way. We had about half a dozen beds in the RAP which we used for the sick who needed to be closely monitored for a day or two. If they needed further attention, we sent them to the hospital, which was located nearby in Roberts Barracks. (Our regiment was not isolated: we were still part of the 8th Division with access to a casualty clearing station, a general hospital — fully equipped, with 500 to 1000 beds — and a field ambulance.) I insisted that a sick parade be treated as a parade: the men had to assemble in order, no straggling and no nonsense. Maintaining order and discipline would be essential for survival.

With all our men together for the first time since action commenced, I took the opportunity to conduct a complete medical inspection. One by one, each man visited the RAP so I could examine his skin for signs of wounds or diseases, in addition to what was known as the 'short-arm' parade, where I checked for signs of venereal disease (syphilis, gonorrhoea and other sexually transmitted diseases). Among military men, there have been a lot of jokes told about such inspections, and numerous cartoons have been drawn of an RMO sitting with his cap over his eyes, looking towards the nether regions of men, and uttering: 'Morning Jones, Morning Smith.'

Sick parades and medical inspections gave me the chance to know my men as individuals. I can only liken it to a cow cocky who really knows his herd — who can say, 'Gee, Daisy doesn't look too good today' from a hundred yards. Regular examinations enabled me to develop a very specific knack for knowing when someone really needed a visit to the doctor, even if he wasn't willing to go on parade.

One of the first rulings the IJA handed down to us in captivity was that we were to wind our watches forward. While the sun still rose and set at the usual time, we were ordered to live on 'Tokyo Time' and we learned to begin our mornings in darkness. We were also instructed to convert from using the imperial system of measurement to metric. Neither of these demands proved too taxing, but adjusting to a radically changed diet proved difficult for all of us.

In theory, our daily prisoner-of-war ration scale per man was: 500 grams rice; 50 grams meat; 50 grams flour; 100 grams vegetables; 15 grams milk; 20 grams sugar; 5 grams salt; 5 grams tea; 5 grams oil and, in addition, there was to be an issue of 40 cigarettes per man per month. I calculated that the ration provided 2000 calories per day plus an additional 500 calories from 'extras' (such as cheese, dried fruit, ham and fish) — if they ever eventuated. In practice, we received far, far less and when our own surplus supplies of rations ran out many of the men found themselves experiencing real hunger for the first time.

It was a dramatic change from our accustomed Australian ration, which provided over 3000 calories, including up to 500 grams of meat with potatoes, bread, butter, cheese, vegetables and fruit. Then there was the additional problem of learning how to cook rice. Initially, with the absence of salt, the men found the rice unpalatable, so Division Headquarters, with Japanese permission, authorised working parties to visit a beach nearby to collect sea water in tins and drums. The men built billycarts from salvaged timber, axles and wheels so they could drag the heavy tins and drums back to camp. The cooks experimented to find an acceptable ratio of sea water to fresh water to satisfy the troops. They did a sterling job considering none of us really knew how we wanted the rice: dry, soft, moist or even as a baked rice pudding, just 'like Mother used to make'. Before long they developed a technique of bashing the rice on a hard surface to make flour and then advanced to making pastries, biscuits, buns and flapjacks.

About a week or so into our time at Changi rumours started to circulate of a Japanese massacre at Alexandra Hospital, a British military hospital in Singapore. Word had it that only hours before Allied surrender, Japanese troops had charged through the grounds of the hospital and killed a British officer who was waving a white flag at them. Working their way from room to room they bayoneted victims without prejudice: doctors, nurses and patients — even those lying on operating tables. We had long suspected what our enemy was capable of, so acts of violence were not surprising, but to hear of such brutality so close to our new home, and to women and the sick, made us realise that any threats made by our keepers were likely to be fair dinkum. This news made all of us angry — as well as frustrated: it further highlighted how helpless we now were to retaliate. We were confined men who could do little more than speculate as to our own future. We thought we had experienced hell during the last week of the Malayan campaign, but we were still to realise that there were many depths of hell under the control of the Japanese, and each would be worse than the last.

IN EARLY MARCH, TOGETHER with most of the units of the 22nd and 27th Brigades AIF, we moved from Birdwood Camp to

Selarang Barracks, which was still home to Division Headquarters. Selarang Barracks featured a large square parade ground surrounded by concrete buildings, but living conditions were still primitive — and crowded. We had to squeeze more than 700 men into a building that had previously held 120, stacking *charpoys* (wooden-framed beds with rope strung across to form a quasi-mattress) on top of each other to create multistorey bunks. Our beds harboured masses of bugs, which were murderous during the night. Many of the men preferred sleeping on the concrete floor.

Attendance at my daily sick parade averaged about 30 to 40, including two cases of dysentery. Other units which were less strict with hygiene reported up to 50 per cent down with dysentery. Beriberi, a disease due to a prolonged deficiency in vitamin B1, was also becoming a problem, initially apparent in the form of swelling of the lower limbs, the abdomen and, to a lesser extent, the face. In an improvised effort to treat beriberi, I sent special parties of men out to collect hibiscus leaves to add to our meagre and vitamin-deficient rations. As an added incentive, I told the men these leaves contained vitamins that would maintain their virility for when they returned home.[4] It wasn't necessarily true, but collecting the leaves gave them a job to do.

It didn't take long for many of our men to realise that with Japanese guards rarely present and no physical walls surrounding our camp, there was very little other than fear keeping any of us 'imprisoned'. The Japanese knew there was nowhere to which we could escape. Our Anglo-Saxon appearance in an Asian country ensured none of us stood a decent chance of fleeing captivity unnoticed. During the night, some of the more daring of our men started slipping through the wire boundary which surrounded our camp to trade with local Malays and Chinese. Hungry men swapped their watches and pens and other personal possessions for eggs, tins of milk, meat, fruit and other foodstuffs. A black market quickly flourished.

Whenever I could take a break from work I maintained in earnest the diary I had commenced during action. The Japanese only ever arrived at our quarters on official inspections, and always accompanied by Division Headquarters staff, so I didn't have to worry about guards sneaking up on me. Still, I was careful only to log basic facts. I avoided references to anything which might incriminate me or anyone else should my jottings ever fall into the wrong hands. I resisted embellishment, hoping that the key words and phrases I recorded would be enough to trigger my memory at a later date.

To conceal and protect my diary, I set about making a waterproof wallet. I remained thankful we had arrived at Changi with all of our gear, including our anti-gas kits. I unpacked my gas cape, a poncho made from a waxy water-resistant material, and cut out two small rectangular pieces. Then I stitched together a pouch with a fold-over flap using cotton drawn through candle wax. Inside I kept my Army pay book, my photo of my cousin Pat and my diary notebook. I carried it at all times in either my shirt or trouser pocket.

BY APRIL THE JAPANESE were sending working parties of POWs from Changi to Singapore, to work on both the docks and the construction of a Japanese memorial to honour the 2000 or more killed at Bukit Timah. Within a month only about 5000 Australians remained in camp.[5] In early May, Division Headquarters was ordered by the Japanese to select a force of 3000 men for an 'overseas party' — destination not stated. Wild and varied rumours flew thick and fast around the camp. (Rumours, by then, had become a currency of their own. In captivity, information was always at a premium, and where there is demand, there is always supply.) There was talk of a Red Cross ship coming to repatriate us; of our moving to a convalescent camp — Borneo was only one of the many countries bandied around; or of being sent on some sort of working party. Others wanted to believe we were to be exchanged for Japanese prisoners of war being held by Allied forces.

Major General Boots Callaghan, now in command of the 8th Division AIF following the escape of Lieutenant General Gordon Bennett,[6] ordered that the selected force of 3000 was to consist of three battalions, each of 1000 men, so composed that if the group was ever released, it would be able to fight as a brigade. It was to be known as 'A' Force — the first force to leave Singapore.

Brigadier Arthur Varley was to be in overall command of this new force. No. 1 Battalion was to be commanded by Lieutenant Colonel George Ramsay and made up mainly of infantry; No. 2 Battalion was to be commanded by Lieutenant Colonel Charles Anderson[7] and made up of specialist units such as artillery, engineers, signallers, and half a casualty clearing station; while No. 3 Battalion was to be commanded by Major Charles Green and consist mainly of infantry and machine-gunners. With this plan in place, Division Headquarters sent out orders to each of the existing brigades and their associated units to provide men for each battalion. (Each battalion would come to be known as Ramsay Force, Anderson Force and Green Force respectively.)

There were mixed feelings amongst the men, depending on which rumour they believed. Some really wanted to be selected while others didn't mind, as long as they could stick with their mates. Some volunteered but most waited for orders. There is an old army saying: 'never volunteer'; only go wherever you are ordered — the belief being that if you try to control your own destiny, it will rarely work in your favour. I chose to wait. Initially, the RMO of the 2/10th Field Regiment had been nominated, but he became ill a few days prior to departure and I was ordered to become RMO of No. 2 Battalion.

On my final night at Changi, I was treated to a 'Last Supper' of eggs, tomatoes and cheese, purchased on the black market, with the CO John Wright, 2 i/c John Workman, and mates Stuart

Ward, Theo Walker, Des Makepeace and Frank Ball. We attempted to celebrate over dinner, but the mood was sombre: of this group, only Stuart Ward and I had been selected for 'A' Force. Most of us had been together since November 1940 — and I had been mates with Des since we were boys — so the impending separation of our close-knit group was difficult. I was fortunate that two of my medical orderlies, Jim Armstrong and Pinkey Rhodes, would be joining me as my RAP staff members, along with two others, Don Booth and Arthur Baker. Des and I exchanged humorous quips and promised each other that whoever made it home first would tell the other's family he was alive and well in May 1942. We accepted our fate in the way we were expected to as trained soldiers; crack-hardy men.

Before going to bed that night, I packed a stash of my personal medical supplies in my kit bag and refilled my hipflask with brandy from some secret stores within the camp. I went to sleep hopeful that better days lay ahead: nearly all of us were inveterate optimists, and at this point, a happy ending still didn't seem out of the question. Life in captivity wasn't yet terrible and I suspect that my experiences at Changi might not match the expectations of many readers. The name 'Changi' has, in recent times, somehow come to embody the misery and suffering of POW existence. For me, Changi will always be remembered as a virtual paradise, a place where we were largely left to our own devices, free from the brutality of guards and with access to some food, water and medical supplies. Following action, our brief stay at Changi was a relative reprieve. While captivity preyed on our minds, the deprivations and hardships we experienced throughout our months there were not particularly severe or difficult to endure in comparison to what was to follow. My time there was spent in limbo, slowly coming to terms with my new status as a prisoner of war. Changi was merely a holding pen before we were farmed out into a new way of life: Railway life.

CHAPTER SIX

'A' FORCE
Changi to Thanbyuzayat
May–September 1942

Three thousand prisoners of war squatted on the bomb-damaged wharves of the Singapore docks, staring at two small cargo ships. Even the most idealistic among us could only describe them as rust buckets. One was about 8000 tonnes in size, the other just 5000 tonnes: they looked not much larger than the Manly ferries back home. It was impossible to comprehend how so many men would cram onboard such sorry-looking ships, or that they were even seaworthy.

It was only mid-morning but the temperature was already rocketing, our dirty uniforms clammy against hot skin. We had been up since 0530, ready to be paraded in the grounds of Changi for the final time before being packed into trucks for the first leg of our journey. Upon arrival at the wharves, the Japanese had ordered some of our men to unload heavy sacks of rice from the trucks down onto the docks. The rest of us had nothing to do but sit on baked concrete and wait; it was a new lesson in patience. For many, today was our first direct interaction with the guards, most of whom were privates. Dressed in the green uniform of the Imperial Japanese Army — loose shirts, breeches with puttees and split-toe canvas boots — each guard was armed with a rifle and bayonet, and carried a length of bamboo or timber. They looked eager to assert their authority. 'No Smoking' signs had been hung along the wharves but many of our men lit up nonetheless, to pass the time and take their minds off the heat. The consequences were immediate. Sour-faced guards delivered bashings ranging from a brutal slap across the face and a bamboo whipping to a hammer on the head with a piece of timber. Anger rose inside me, but there was nothing any of us could do but watch. When the guards backed off, Jim Armstrong and I moved amongst the crowd, cleaning and dressing bloody lacerations to the faces and heads of the beaten men.

In the early afternoon, most of us sunburned and all of us restless from the interminable wait, we were finally ordered to board the ships: 2000 (including me) on the slightly larger vessel, the *Toyohasi Maru*, and the remaining 1000 on the *Celebes Maru*. Neither ship displayed the Red Cross nor any other sign to indicate they were carrying prisoners of war. We were herded like sheep up a narrow loading ramp, guards prodding us with the butts of their rifles.

The majority of men were forced down into the holds, while officers and those who couldn't squeeze below were allowed to stay topside. I made camp with a group of officers beneath a lifeboat on deck: it offered scant protection from the rain that was soon drumming down, but we were much better off than those trapped below. The holds had been remodelled to accommodate the physically smaller Japanese troops and in between the multi-layered platforms there was no more than a metre or so of headroom. Our men crawled on all fours in the darkness trying to find a place to crouch. Jammed in like battery-caged hens, they had no room to move, no light and very little air to breathe. Both above and below deck rats ran riot during the night and the stench of vomit and diarrhoea emanating from the holds was unmistakeable. These vessels deserved their ensuing tag of 'hell ships'.

I established an RAP, of sorts, up on deck — essentially just me standing next to my open medical pannier. Diarrhoea and dysentery were major problems but I only had limited amounts of sulpha drugs (specific treatment for bacillary dysentery) and emetine (for the rarer form of amoebic dysentery). I knew if I administered full treatment for all cases our supplies would fast become exhausted, so I rationed the dosages, issuing short, even token, courses to those who needed them most. In retrospect, this could be considered as a waste of precious supplies, at least in medical terms, but in reality this wasn't the case. When I gave medicine to sick men, it had a psychosomatic effect: it boosted their morale because they felt as though they were being 'treated'. Their ensuing optimism undoubtedly aided their recovery: men who genuinely believed they would get well had a much better chance of making it than those who became negative or lost hope. On a philosophical level, I believed the essential factors in whether a man would survive or not were, first and above all else, his ability to maintain hope and, second, the degree to which he could adapt.

The constant need for the latrine at least gave the men in the holds an opportunity for a breath of fresh air up on deck. With only two five-hole latrines slung over the side of the ship to cater for all of us, the queues were permanent. Our daily diet of a little rice, thin watery stew, tea and one small tin of M&V (meat and vegetables), which had to be shared between 27 men per day (about a tablespoon full each), didn't help matters.

Aside from the miserable conditions onboard, one memory stands out above all others. A few days into our voyage, a group of five men discreetly approached the RAP and formed a semicircle around me. In a quiet voice one of them said, 'Here Doc,' and handed over a large stack of containers of Atebrin. 'These belong to you.' The men had dug up supplies of the malaria drug which had been buried by Division Headquarters at Changi. I held their offering in my arms, speechless. That they were prepared to take such a risk was testament to their support and respect, and I felt honoured to have gained their loyalty.

Their act of defiance was not only heart warming, but also an indication that the morale of our men was slowly being restored. Initial feelings of disappointment and relief over surrender had, by this time, turned to anger about our status as prisoners of war. Denied the opportunity to perform as fighting troops, our men had started to look for different types of victories, against both the Japanese and our own Division Headquarters. Sabotaging our weapons and vehicles, sneaking through the camp's wire at night to trade, and now handing over the Atebrin — these acts all marked the beginning of small but important triumphs: it was our own way of saying we might be down but we're far from out. In captivity, the smallest of wins could create the greatest of joys.

AS WE SAILED ALONG the coast of Burma (today known as Myanmar), we passed lovely emerald green islands and dense jungle lining the shores of the mainland. From a distance, Burma looked very handsome, the kind of land I had imagined travelling to as a boy. None of us had dreamed of exploring the world as prisoners of war, but that didn't stop us from marvelling at nature's brilliance; it was the chance for a brief escape from the reality of our existence. Such memories of beauty have never left me; they remain stored as a collection of unspoiled postcards in my mind.

The initial plan to keep our 3000-strong brigade group intact was thwarted when five days into our voyage the convoy stopped at Victoria Point, on the extreme southern tip of Burma. Here,

Green Force was ordered by the Japanese to disembark, along with two doctors — Captain Claude Anderson and Captain John Higgin — whom Brigadier Varley had insisted join Green Force. Three days later, the convoy arrived at Mergui, on the coast of Burma, where Ramsay Force was ordered by the Japanese to disembark and, again on orders from Varley, half of the casualty clearing staff from Anderson Force also disembarked.[1] Finally, after two more days at sea, the rest of Anderson Force (myself included) arrived at Simbin anchorage, some 40 kilometres from the town of Tavoy.

The Japanese brought barges up to the side of our ship and then provided us with rope ladders fitted with rotting wooden steps. The barges were a good three to four metres drop from the ships' deck and, to add to our troubles, the wind was howling and the sky had opened up to the streaming of rain. The barges rose upwards with the swell, banging against the side of the ship — sometimes breaking one of the wooden steps of the ladder in the process — and then crashed down again. The trick was to climb a little way down the ladder, wait for the swell to bring the barge upwards and then jump backwards, like skydivers, carrying all our worldly possessions on our backs. It was sheer madness, but we had no choice. God only knows how no man was injured.

We spent that night in the Simbin rice godown (warehouse), attempting to sleep on top of rice bags in the company of weevils, fleas and rats. The next morning we rose early to begin the long march to Tavoy, in south-eastern Burma. I started the journey in the front row alongside three other officers. We marched for periods of up to about an hour at a time, with halts in between, passing through lush green paddy fields and paddocks at Simbin village, where we watched horses and cattle grazing and noted the beginning of what seemed to be an infinite string of shrines and Buddhas. Miniature bells tinkled in the hot breeze. At each break my RAP staff — Jim Armstrong, Pinkey Rhodes, Don Booth and

Arthur Baker — helped me attend to the men, applying bandages and what little else we could offer from our own personal kits. The Japanese guards had ordered me to leave my pannier onboard the ship, to be transported by them along with equipment for the casualty clearing station and Battalion Headquarters at a later date. It was proving to be a near impossible task to practise medicine without medicine.

During many of the halts, native Burmese dressed in colourful sarongs ventured out of their bamboo huts to offer us cups of hot water — which was surprisingly refreshing — as well as fruit and biscuit-like pastries. They smiled warmly as they presented us with their gifts, bowing their heads. Their kindness was touching.

Not long into the march, I received word that one of our men had collapsed from exhaustion at the rear of our column. I turned around and made my way back to attend to him as best I could and then returned to my position in the front line. If I'd had any sense I would have stayed at the back from the beginning, because soon after I received another call to the back line. And so it went on for the rest of the march: backwards and forwards between the sick and fatigued men of Anderson Force. With such limited supplies, sometimes the only treatment I could offer was to carry a man's pack for a bit and have a chat to pass some time with his mind otherwise occupied.

After almost eleven hours of gruelling marching, when many of the men were having extreme trouble keeping pace, a guard gave one of our men a particularly forceful prod with his fixed bayonet. I was helping a man nearby and my instinctive and thoughtless reaction was to knock the fixed bayonet out of the guard's hands. I couldn't believe what I had done. The rifle and bayonet lay on the ground nearby. The guard looked stunned. I kept my mouth shut, held my breath and waited for a beating, but the guard quietly reclaimed his weapon and let the incident pass without comment. Maybe it was because he was just as exhausted as we were, or possibly my position of RMO engendered some form of respect from the low-ranked guard; regardless, I escaped retribution. Our keepers, I was discovering, were consistently inconsistent in their punishments.

SHORTLY BEFORE MIDNIGHT WE finally arrived at Tavoy Gaol, where we were issued with our first meal since breakfast — rice, pork and vegetables — and then ordered to resume marching, bound for the Tavoy aerodrome nearby. I persuaded some of the guards to allow men who were too sick or weak to march any further to be carried in the ration trucks, which were following us. I spoke very limited Japanese, picked up from listening to our guards, but together with hand and facial gestures I was able to make myself understood (after all, my parents had taught me the value of sign language). By this stage I was beginning to grasp the Japanese concept of 'loss of face'. Bill Drower, a British officer attached to 'A' Force as an interpreter, was very knowledgeable in regard to Japanese customs and habits; he indoctrinated us to be careful never to put a guard in a position where he would feel humiliated and thereby 'lose face'. We started to realise that we could argue, bargain and persuade, as long as we made sure the guard involved felt he could preserve his pride in the process. It was an art I strived to perfect.

We marched on in torrential rain, our boots gummy with thick mud. One of the men in our battalion calculated I had walked at least double the distance of others due to my to-ing and fro-ing between men collapsing in the lines, and I was definitely feeling the effects. I struggled at the rear of the column, willing my deadened legs to keep moving as we approached the grounds of the aerodrome. It was a toss-up as to who was more buggered: me or the guard plodding by my side. By the time we approached the main gate to the aerodrome, I was just starting to trail behind the guard when out of the darkness I heard a group of Australian voices shout: 'Don't let that little bastard beat you!' Smiling, I pulled myself together and 'sprinted' to the finish line, beating the guard by no more than a nose. It had been a case of one man out-stumbling the other but our blokes counted it as another small win, nonetheless. I can still hear them cheering, 'Good on you, Doc!' Totally spent after our fifteen-hour march, the guard couldn't have cared less.

We crossed the aerodrome and shuffled our way towards a large hangar that was to be our accommodation. Walter Moore, a captain from our regiment, kindly carried my pack. With the weight removed my feet tingled and I experienced the most remarkable sensation of walking on air. It was now 0230, the rain was still pelting down and the guards persisted in counting us numerous times — over and over, finding it impossible to arrive at the correct figure — before allowing us inside our new lodgings. This constant counting was a new frustration to us, but in time we would accept it as standard practice.

The ground inside the hangar was covered in large jagged rocks; it was impossible to clear a smooth surface on which we could lie. Most of us were so physically shattered we fell asleep regardless of the sharp edges jutting into our rain-soaked skin. I was wakened the following afternoon by the sound of more heavy rain belting loudly on the tin roof. Men stripped off and ran outside to enjoy their first wash since leaving Changi.

PRIOR TO THE MALAYAN campaign, the RAF had been building the aerodrome at Tavoy: it was now going to be our job to finish building it for the Japanese (with help from fellow British and Dutch POWs, who had by now joined us from Sumatra). The following day I accompanied Brigadier Varley to the 'hospital' to formally admit the sick according to a pro forma provided by the Japanese. The so-called hospital consisted of timber huts with holes in the wall serving as windows. The huts were in quite good condition but we had no facilities or supplies other than what was left in our own packs. The Japanese dumped 92 of our men at the hospital with no food, no water and no guards. Because our key casualty clearing station staff had not yet arrived from Simbin, I was ordered to look after the hospital in the interlude before they rejoined us. By the time they arrived four days later I had admitted 199 Australians and approximately 130 Dutch.

A total of 250 of our men were progressively sent over 150 kilometres north to the town of Ye to perform bridge work and road repairs, while the rest began construction on the aerodrome. Men on the aerodrome were ordered to dig soil from built-up areas nearby and carry it onto the airstrip to fill deep gullies. They laboured in groups of three: one equipped with a *chunkal* (similar to an oversized hoe), while the other two worked with a bamboo pole and a bag that served as a makeshift bucket. The digger shovelled soil into the bag, which the carriers then tied to the middle of the bamboo pole; they rested the pole across their shoulders and carried the load in tandem, one behind the other, down to the airstrip. Some of the soil was also shifted with assistance from skips on a light rail track, but most was by 'bag and pole'. It was slow and back-breaking work but the men of 'A' Force retained their humour. Finding ways to surreptitiously outwit the guards was their favourite pastime, and it was wonderful for maintaining morale. The Japanese used pegs to mark the area of soil each trio was responsible for digging, and the men took great delight in moving the pegs closer together while guards weren't looking. In retrospect, it might seem childish — playing games with their keepers — but many of our men were in fact not much older than boys, and petty victories were the only ones on offer.

Officers were not required to undertake physical labour: the existing military establishment of rank and command was maintained. Officers were responsible for the administration of the camp and organising and protecting the men, often copping bashings in the process of trying to negotiate better conditions. We were also answerable to the Japanese in fulfilling the daily quotas demanded for work parties. In Anderson Force, the men didn't resent officers for not having to do physical work; they were grateful to have a buffer between themselves and the Japanese. This absence of resentment was largely due to the fact that Brigadier Varley and Colonel Anderson were adamant that officers were not to receive significant privileges over the men (for example, increased food rations) and the men greatly respected them for this.

After two days of monotonous work on the aerodrome, we were moved from the hangar into timber huts that had been constructed by the RAF. We had ample room here and the smooth wooden floors were considered heavenly by all. Two huts were allocated to each company, along with separate kitchens. Before long the men had made mud ovens for the cooks and converted 44-gallon drums into pots. Our casualty clearing station and Battalion Headquarters equipment arrived soon after, including my medical pannier, which had been looted of everything aside from my syringe and bottles of Ringer's solution (a saline mixture with minerals added, used to aid hydration). I formally protested to the Japanese, requesting to have the items replaced, but it was a waste of breath.

Our loss of medical supplies quickly led to a spate of deaths at Tavoy. The first occurred the same day work began on the aerodrome. It was a Dutchman and his death was probably due to dysentery. The first AIF death followed the next day, definitely from dysentery, and six more succumbed the day after. Without medicine, there was little I could do to stop the ravages of this disease apart from making sure ill men received what little food was available, and negotiating with the guards to let them rest and avoid physical labour.

It proved to be a week of senseless deaths when only 24 hours later eight men caught attempting to escape were summarily shot. News of their violent execution without trial rocked us all. Inside Japanese Headquarters, Brigadier Varley, at great personal risk, had reportedly threatened a Japanese officer in a last-ditch attempt to fight for the lives of his men, announcing that following the end of the war he would personally see to it that the Japanese officers involved would be tried before an international court on a charge of murder.[2]

The Japanese held no regard for the Geneva or Hague Conventions — or any other international rules of warfare — so Varley's efforts were wasted. Our captors wanted to make it clear that the death penalty for attempted escape was no idle threat. Varley, Colonel Anderson, Captain Drower and Padre Bashford were the only witnesses to the eight men being gunned down by a firing squad. Rumours swept through camp that the escapees had been forced to dig their own graves before being shot.

We were livid, but there was damn all we could do about it. We had lost fifteen men from 'A' Force in three days, and all of the deaths were preventable had it not been for the cruelty of our keepers. These losses deepened our understanding of the reality of our lives as prisoners of war, and made it blatantly clear that the optimistic notions of possible repatriation or being exchanged for Japanese prisoners held by Allied troops were false. This was our life now, and we would have to turn our anger into determination if we were going to survive.

BY THE BEGINNING OF June we were well settled into our living quarters and had managed to obtain tables and stools adjacent to our sleeping bags and beds. The view from our window was always engaging, especially at sunrise and sunset when the sky was lit with a wide array of colours that reflected onto the hills in the background. The aerodrome overlooked a paddy valley and the picturesque hills; under other circumstances it would have been a pleasant place to visit.

Work on the aerodrome was nowhere near complete but the Japanese decided the airstrip was ready to be trialled. We were ordered to line the runway to watch the auspicious event alongside the very excited guards. With our heads tilted back, all eyes on the sky, the plane descended, luminous against the burning sun. Suddenly, an Australian voice cried out: 'Crash you bastard, crash.' His lone chant quickly developed into a chorus: 'Crash you bastard, crash. Crash you bastard, crash. Crash you bastard, crash . . .' It grew louder as the plane neared land. The guards ignored us, their eyes still clapped on their man in the sky.

The wheels hit the airstrip and the plane thumped and bounced along the dirt before flipping over and crashing. We could scarcely believe our eyes. The chanting ceased. The plane was a complete wreck. As the pilot climbed from the cockpit, apparently unharmed, we roared madly — another notch in our collective belt. The guards were silent, their eyes looking towards the ground. No doubt the pilot would be punished for causing such a grave loss of face.

In captivity, a man's sense of right and wrong can quickly change. With a mentality of 'us and them', we did not hesitate to will bad luck and suffering upon our keepers. We were at their mercy 24 hours a day, enduring slave labour, and thoughts of retribution and the cruel fate of our captors became a pastime in which nearly all prisoners of war engaged.

We were surprised not to be punished for our disobedient cheering, and even more surprised the following day to receive three letter cards to send back to our homelands. The cards, issued by the IJA, were highly censored once back in Japanese hands, so there was little we could convey, but we hoped they would reach home and give our families comfort that we were still very much alive. I sent one to my mother, one to Arthur and Linda at Kyogle and one to the Martins, our neighbours in Summer Hill. On the same day a party of 200 more Dutch, both Holland Dutch and Indonesian Dutch, arrived in camp to assist with the remaining aerodrome work. Among them was Lieutenant Pfeiffer, a language professor from a Dutch university. He gave me daily lessons in classical Dutch so I could conduct a sick parade with minimal assistance from an interpreter, to save time.

The relationship between different nationalities of prisoners of war within camps was cautiously friendly. The Brits, by and large, we plain didn't like: we resented being looked down upon as their poor colonial cousins, and continued to be dismayed by their lax approach to hygiene, as well as their insistence on maintaining hierarchical structures at all times. We found many of their officers to be unbearably pompous and ever-willing to demand special privileges at the expense of their own men. We got along with the Dutch far better, particularly the indigenous Indonesian and Eurasian Dutch (as opposed to the Holland Dutch). They had even more to learn about hygiene than the Brits, but they were always friendly and particularly good at selecting leaves in the wild to add to our meagre and mostly meat-free and vitamin-deficient rations. Despite our differences, all prisoners of war were united in the common goal of staying alive.

In the township of Tavoy the RAF had established a library consisting of a large range of books, from encyclopaedias to popular novels. Brigadier Varley conned the Japanese into allowing us to distribute the books as toilet paper, using the explanation that palm leaves were becoming abrasive on tender bottoms. Each man was issued with three or four books which, in effect, became part of a mobile lending library. After the initial rush to read the salacious *Lady Chatterly's Lover* by D.H. Lawrence, the most popular genres were poetry, philosophy, classic novels and encyclopaedias. The Bible was also in demand, not so much for its spiritual content but rather its thin paper, which was ideal for rolling cigarettes with chopped up cigars as tobacco.

Sunday was a rest day: church parades were held in the morning and concerts at night, much to the enjoyment of the troops — and even the guards. Quizzes conducted around the campfire at night were also popular. The encyclopaedias were used to help formulate questions and check answers. We assembled in teams led by various quiz masters, all of whom took it very seriously. Quiz activity extended into the field, too. In the working groups of three, the man on the *chunkal* would pose a question — for example, who won the Melbourne Cup in 1903? — and the two carriers would then discuss possible answers on their way to dump the soil before returning to offer their final response. It helped to pass the time and keep their minds busy: our minds were the only thing over which we could still maintain control.

My closest mates at Tavoy were medical orderlies Jim Armstrong and Pinkey Rhodes, as well as Major Don Kerr (2 i/c of Anderson Force) and Major John Shaw (in command of the engineers of Anderson Force). When we had free time, we passed the hours playing contract bridge using a pack of well-worn cards or having long discussions. We refought the war several times and debated whether or not Lieutenant General Gordon Bennett had been right to escape following the surrender.

At the end of June we were very excited to receive our first pay: 10 cents per day for privates, 15 for NCOs and 25 for warrant officers, with pay issued once a month. We could only assume our captors decided to pay us so we could purchase food from local Burmese traders — ensuring that the Japanese received a cut of the takings in the process. Brigadier Varley and Colonel Anderson made sure that all officers received the same rate of pay as the warrant officers. From our pay was deducted 10, 15, and 20 per cent respectively to be pooled in a Red Cross fund, with monies used to buy food for the sick. (Don Murchison was the International Red Cross representative attached to 'A' Force, and he administered the fund.) In addition, the Japanese deducted a significant sum for our 'board and lodging'. Whatever was left over was ours to spend. The Japanese occupation notes were small, like Monopoly money, and branded with 'The Japanese Government'; they were based on the Burmese currency of cents and rupees. We called it Mickey Mouse money. The main Burmese trader was nicknamed 'Ali Baba' and the guards encouraged his visits to our camp. The cooks were already making bread rolls, pastries, fish cakes, rissoles and pap (very soft boiled ground rice), and with new supplies from Ali Baba we were soon enjoying dried peas, beans and fish, as well as jam from pineapples, ginger, limes, *chindegar* (sugar) and molasses.

Like Changi, I remember Tavoy as a time of relative plenty. Despite the appalling journey on the hell ships, the theft of medical supplies and the loss of our men, life wasn't yet unbearable — and the health of our men had actually improved significantly. I still have a copy of the original medical statistics I recorded daily in the form of graphs and tables. At Tavoy, the number on sick parade fell from 40 per cent in the middle of June to 30 per cent by the beginning of July, 20 per cent by the middle of July and to less than 10 per cent by September. With access to pay and Ali Baba, and Red Cross purchases for the sick, day-to-day survival became manageable. The whole period was a good example of what could be achieved simply through a better diet and living conditions, despite hard physical labour. The better the health of the men, the more physical work they were able to perform. It seemed logical that our keepers might also see the benefit of keeping us fed and clean — but in days to come we would realise that logic had nothing to do with whether men lived or died.

THE DAYS DRAGGED BY and by the end of September work on the aerodrome was complete and we were ordered to march to Tavoy wharf, some five kilometres distant. One thousand of us waited to be loaded onto four 100-tonne barges, and two six-metre launches which were also used to tow the barges. The walls of the barges were about five metres high and in the excessive heat many men suffered salt deficiency cramps. The Japanese could not fit all of us on board, so almost 300 of our men were ordered back to Tavoy. That night we were transferred onto the *Unkai Maru* — a tramp steamer of approximately 1000 tonnes — and we sailed the next morning. We were given dry rations, tea and one bottle of water per man per day. Smoking was forbidden and, with the full knowledge of what the consequences would be for doing otherwise, we obeyed. There were only two latrines for more than 700 of us.

After 28 hours' sailing we arrived at Moulmein, south of the ancient city of Thaton, on 1 October. The next morning we travelled by train to Thanbyuzayat, about 55 kilometres away. Loaded onto hot and dusty rail wagons, we passed time admiring the magnificent scenery of Burma: gigantic teak trees, growing densely together, formed much of the landscape and reminded me of my Kyogle and Cougal days.

In camp at Thanbyuzayat, we expected life to remain the same as it had been at Tavoy, but then one morning it became apparent that radical changes were afoot. On our third day at Thanbyuzayat we were ordered on parade early in the morning. Japanese Headquarters informed us that our Army establishment of battalions and companies was to be replaced immediately by Japanese *kumis*, consisting of 50 men each. Each *kumi* was to be led by a *kumicho* (a position usually held by a lieutenant); with a *hancho* (held by a captain) in charge of two *kumis*. Furthermore, parades were to be called *tenkos*, and during every *tenko* we would be required to 'number off' in Japanese — '*ichi* [one], *ni* [two], *san* [three],' and so on — down the line. Even the bugle calls were to be played Japanese-style. Each prisoner of war was allocated a wooden token with a unique POW number engraved on one side as a means of identification: I was to be known as number 1912. We were all now members of the No. 3 Thai POW camp,[3] of which Lieutenant Colonel Yoshitada Nagatomo was the commander.

Nagatomo was a small, cocky man, immaculately turned out, who carried a Samurai sword on his left side. We stood on parade in the sun for over three hours while he delivered a seemingly never-ending manifesto in Japanese, with another guard translating his words into English for us. Life, it seemed, was going to be cheap: the penalty for being sick would be half-rations, and, as we were already well aware, the sentence for attempted escape was death. Towards the end of his address he announced that we would be working on a railway:

> At the time of such shortness of materials, your lives are preserved by the Military and all of you must reward them with your labour. By the hand of Nippon Army, railway works to connect Thailand [Siam] and Burma have started, to the great interest of the world. There are deep jungles where no man comes to clear them by cutting the trees. There is [sic] also countless difficulties and sufferings, but you shall have the honour to join in this great work which was never done before, and you should do your best efforts . . .[4]

In conclusion, Nagatomo raised his neatly coiffed head from his script and proffered a final piece of advice: 'Work cheerfully, and from henceforth you shall be guided by this motto.'

After working on the aerodrome at Tavoy the men viewed the railway work ahead as simply more of the same: slave labour, but nothing they couldn't conquer. We were all extremely hot, bored to tears and dead tired after standing in the heat for so long. We were neither impressed nor alarmed by Nagatomo's words, we just wanted to get out of the sun. None of us had any appreciation of just what we were being led into. Had we suspected the pitiless suffering that lay ahead, I wonder, even now, whether many of us would have chosen the quick way out, rather than lingering on with an ever-decreasing chance of survival.

PART 3

THE BURMA−SIAM RAILWAY

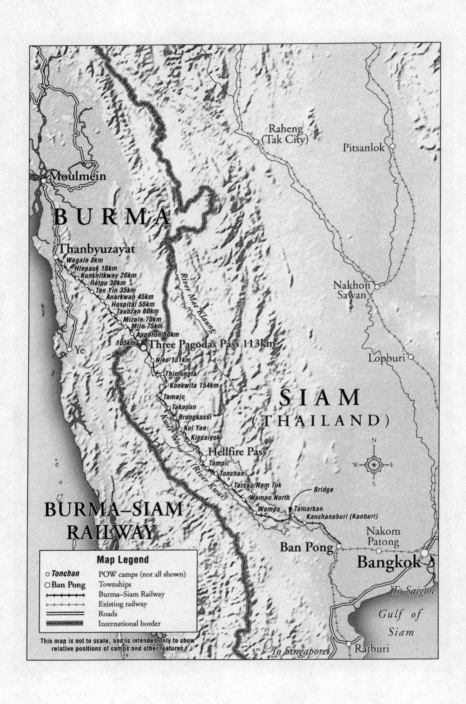

Raheng
(Tak City)

Pitsanlok

Moulmein

B U R M A

Thanbyuzayat
Wegale 8km
Hlepauk 18km
Kunknitkway 26km
Retpu 30km
Tan Yin 35km
Anarkwan 45km
Hospital 55km
Taunzan 60km
Mizale 70km
Milo 75km
Apparon 80km
105km   Three Pagodas Pass 113km
Ye
Nike 131km
Thimongta
Konkwita 154km
Tamajo
Takanun
Brankassi
Kui Yae
Kinsaiyok

River Mae Klaung

Nakhon
Sawan

S I A M
(T H A I L A N D)

Lopburi

Kwai Noi

Hellfire Pass
Tampii
Tonchan
Tarsao/Nam Tok
Wampo North
Wampo
Tamarkan
Kanchanaburi (Kanburi)

Bridge

(River Kwai)

N
W   E
S

BURMA–SIAM
RAILWAY

Ban Pong

Nakom
Patong

Bangkok

To Saigon

Gulf of
Siam

Ratburi

To Singapore

Map Legend

○ *Tonchan*	POW camps (not all shown)
○ **Ban Pong**	Townships
⊢⊢⊢⊢⊢⊢	Burma–Siam Railway
⊦⊦⊦⊦⊦⊦	Existing railway
══════	Roads
━━━━━━	International border

This map is not to scale, and is intended only to show
relative positions of camps and other features

CHAPTER SEVEN

RAILWAY LIFE

Thanbyuzayat (0 Kilo camp) to Hlepauk (18 Kilo camp)
October–December 1942

Swinging from the army belt of every guard was a polished bayonet encased in a metallic scabbard. During our eighteen-kilometre march south-east from Thanbyuzayat to Hlepauk, we watched our keepers unhook these weapons, fix them to their rifles and then felt them stabbing at our bare legs, shouting at us to keep pace. It took us seven long hours to reach our jungle destination on 10 October.

Hlepauk, our first camp along the planned railway route, consisted of huts made of bamboo with *attap* roofs — 100 metres long and divided into 40 bays to hold 270 men. Inside, we slept side by side on platforms raised a couple of feet off the ground; knots in the bamboo slats were sharp against our skin. At either end of the hut there was an opening where guards prowled at random intervals. A Japanese flag in the parade ground fluttered in the muggy breeze. A shorter hut, about 50 metres long, was used for the kitchen, RAP and makeshift hospital. Nearby was a creek which, although dark with mud, provided water we could use in the kitchen and for bathing, or boil for drinking. During the night we became accustomed to strange bedfellows — all sorts of bugs, beetles, hairy grubs and scorpions. The air was thick with mosquitoes droning around our ears and feasting on our sweaty bodies. It would be hard to escape malaria in the jungles of Burma.

Slave gangs consisting of Allied prisoners of war and native conscripts were expected to achieve a near-impossible feat: to build a railway in a remote jungle environment connecting an already established railway network at Thanbyuzayat, in Burma, to another existing network at Bampong, in Siam (Thailand) — effectively creating a Japanese supply line from Burma through to Indo-China. This same overland route had been previously surveyed by the British, who had deemed it impractical due to prohibitive costs, endemic tropical diseases and engineering challenges including teak forest terrain and torrential rainfall (about 10,000 millimetres annually, most of which fell in a four-month period). But with access to slave labour, the Japanese did not share these same concerns. Preparing to mount their offensive in India, they wanted to avoid travelling by ship in exposed waters around the Malayan peninsula, a distance of over 3000 kilometres. The railway, covering a distance of just 400 kilometres, would provide an ideal solution.

While 'A' Force commenced construction on the Burma side, working its way south-east, British and Dutch POWs were being gathered to start working north-west from Bampong, where they would soon be joined by other Australians. Groups of prisoners of war were positioned in camps along the planned route of the Railway to work on specific 'sections', with each camp labelled according to its distance, in kilometres, from Thanbyuzayat (0 Kilo camp).

The men were ordered to continue embankment work, but this time under new rules. The Japanese advised that 0.6 cubic metres of excavation was to be each man's daily work quota and only one day in ten would be allocated for rest. The work, while boring and carried out with primitive tools, was not overly taxing for the relatively fit men: they had few problems achieving their quota. While this was officially the beginning of Railway life, our days even then didn't seem more than we could endure; we remained resolute in our determination to survive this sentence of labour so the rest of our lives could continue — hopefully some time sooner rather than later.

Our first few days at Hlepauk passed without incident. Men carried out their work orders from dawn to just before sunset, guards pacing around them, and I tended to sick men in camp. But by the end of that same week, the Japanese made yet another demand: all prisoners of war were to sign a formal 'no escape' undertaking: 'I the undersigned hereby swear on my honour that I will not under any circumstances attempt to escape.'[1]

Back at Thanbyuzayat, Brigadier Varley, who had remained with our own 'A' Force (Brigade) Headquarters, and other senior officers were refusing to sign. Word reached us that Varley's resistance angered the Japanese so greatly that he and other senior officers involved had been imprisoned in isolation, and ordered not to be released until they complied with their signatures. After days of punishment, including confinement and starvation, Varley conceded, satisfied that his protests would provide sufficient evidence at a later date to prove the undertakings had been signed 'under duress'.

Rumours continued to spread among our camp that men at Thanbyuzayat were autographing the parole using monikers such as 'Mickey Mouse', 'King Kong' and anything else other than their real names. It seemed an appropriate response to such a farcical request: other than inside our own imaginations, there was nowhere to which we could escape.

AFTER ENDURING UNRELENTING RAIN since Tavoy, it suddenly stopped at the end of October. The dry season had arrived. Our men now had to endure working beneath the burning sun wearing no more than shorts and a slouch hat, if they still had them, or a G-string (a loin cloth of scant proportions). On their feet they wore remnant boots, or clogs, hand made in camp from a Dutch-pattern using teak wood for the sole and a strap of webbing hand 'stapled' with bits of wire to hold them on. Most of the men were still having little trouble meeting the work targets set by the Japanese, often working faster than required just so they could finish early and get out of the sun. But our keepers soon took advantage of this, further increasing the required work rate and working hours, and officially marking the onset of persistent '*speedo! speedo!*' (work faster) orders.

My own days entailed conducting sick parades and visiting the sick in our improvised hospital. In the mornings I held a formal sick parade, with numbers averaging 170 to 220 a day, about 35 per cent of camp strength. At lunchtime, a meal was usually sent out to the men on the Railway — baskets of rice and meagre tubs of watery stew — and if anybody had become ill or collapsed during the morning they'd come back to camp with the food carriers and report to me. I still possessed my stethoscope and a thermometer but I rarely used them during sick parades. The diagnosis was usually quite obvious and, if it wasn't, beyond classifying a man 'No Duty' to allow him to escape physical labour for a day or two, there was often not much I could do. In the main, I was seeing ulcers of the lower leg, malaria, beriberi and occasional cases of dengue. Like most RMOs of the AIF, I had no previous knowledge or experience of tropical ulcers. They generally resulted from an initial trauma in the form of a scratch or abrasion, usually courtesy of spiky bamboo, handling a *chunkal* or being hit by flying bits of stone. Infection usually followed and, with malnutrition reducing the ability of a man's body to combat the infection, the abrasion could quickly develop into an ulcer.

When contemplating how to treat the ulcers, my thoughts returned to Uncle Arthur back in Kyogle. I fondly recalled his medical mantra: 'Make every movement count.' Whenever I touched a patient in his presence, Arthur had always insisted there was to be 'No fiddling, Rowley.' With this in mind, it seemed a logical principle to ensure I didn't destroy any healthy tissue when dealing with the ulcers. Along with my orderlies, I placed hot foments on the hard scabs of ulcers to soften them up, then, ever so gently, we used forceps to remove all dead tissue, taking care not to damage the new, pink granulating tissue. It was a painstaking and time-consuming process. We treated three or four men simultaneously, running backwards and forwards between our patients at timed intervals. In total we spent about half an hour treating each ulcer, which we then covered with bandages — improvised from torn sheets, shorts, shirts, mosquito nets and even blankets all sterilised in boiling water. We left the bandages on for four to seven days, to prevent damage to the granulating tissue and ensure minimal handling. Gouging or scraping the ulcers was strictly forbidden.

Cases of pellagra were also appearing. Pellagra, like beriberi, is due to a deficiency in a component of vitamin B, specifically B_{12}. In its initial stages, the effects include inflammation and painful swelling of the tongue, angular stomatitis (inflammation at the angles of the mouth), and a 'butterfly' rash that creates a symmetrical pattern on both sides of a patient's face. The scrotum is also affected, with skin becoming dry, cracked and intensely itchy. Known as 'hot balls' or 'fire balls' by the men, it was an incredibly uncomfortable and painful condition. The cases in camp were only displaying early signs, but it was still a serious concern. Pellagra was also known as 'the four Ds': dermatitis, followed by diarrhoea, then dementia and, finally, death.

With no access to vitamin B_1 to treat beriberi or B_{12} for pellagra, we had to improvise. We attempted to make yeast, known for its high vitamin B content, by fermenting rice and potatoes, and soon succeeded in producing many litres of what we labelled 'brewer's yeast' (in fact, it was wild yeast). The growth of this culture was monitored using my microscope, previously salvaged by Jim Armstrong from an abandoned plantation hospital in Malaya.[2] As with the hibiscus leaves I prescribed in Changi, I was doubtful that this yeast would make any real difference but the men involved in the production were glad to feel useful, and the men drinking it felt as though they were being treated. Without adequate medical supplies it was the best idea I could come up with.

IN NOVEMBER WE WERE introduced to Korean guards (Korea was under Japanese rule between 1910 and the end of the Second World War). The Japanese were still in overall command and governing the construction of the Railway, but the Korean guards were, from herein, by our sides all day every day. The Japanese viewed the Koreans as no more than a low-grade labour force at their disposal, using them as gaolers so they could keep more of their own soldiers fighting in the war. Fuelled by the Japanese, word spread throughout camp that the Korean guards were 'gaol birds' themselves, only released so they could be drafted into the Japanese Army. For once a rumour seemed likely: these new guards looked a crooked bunch to us.

We quickly bestowed nicknames on the new guards. Of particular note was 'Peanut' Tomoto, so named because we thought he had a brain the size of a pea and that he was totally nuts. He was a lean man with a mean face, his beady eyes close together, and he always wore a sneer when he spoke. In broken English he frequently talked about sex in front of us, boasting that when Japan invaded Australia they would also conquer 'Australian girls. *Jiggy-jig.*' His voice was effeminate and from the way he stared at some of our men, many of us soon wondered if his only, or even main, interest was in women.

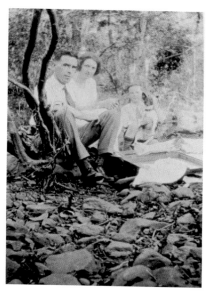

ABOVE Me, aged about thirteen, on a picnic with Aunt Linda and Uncle Arthur at Kyogle.

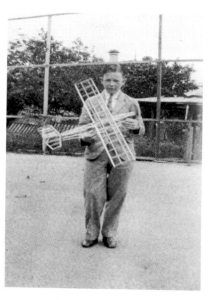

ABOVE Posing on our tennis court with a balsa model aeroplane. I was about fifteen here, and fascinated with how things worked. My family called me 'Little Why'.

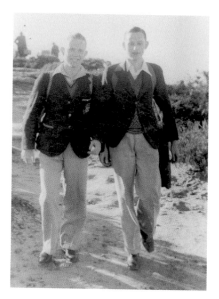

ABOVE Me (left) with my brother, Frank, as teenagers.

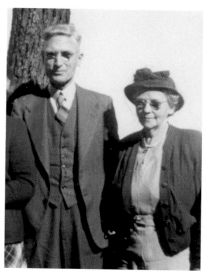

ABOVE My parents, Charles and Clive. This photo was taken in 1952.

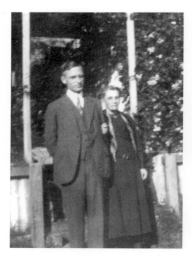

ABOVE Father and Grandmother Polson, circa 1920, outside Guyra.

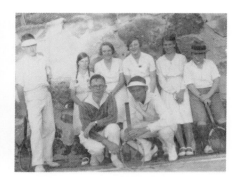

ABOVE Tennis was one of my favourite pastimes as a boy. Here I am pictured (front row, wearing specs) with a group of friends I used to play with at Chatswood, where my good friend Des Makepeace (front row next to me) lived.

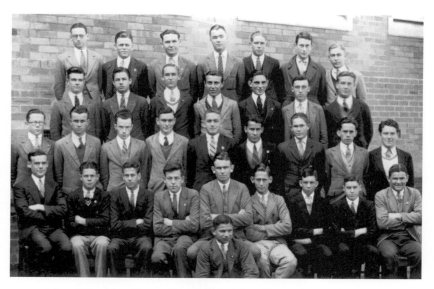

ABOVE Class 5C at Fort Street Boys' High School in Sydney, 1932. I am sixteen years old (third row down, first from the left), with my friend Keith Elphinstone (directly in front of me) and Des Makepeace (five to the right of Keith).

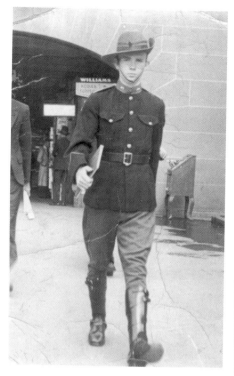

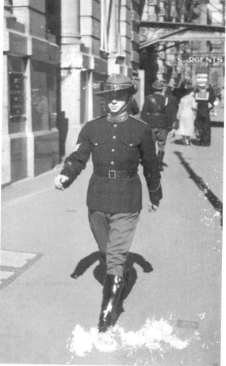

LEFT Me as a gunner, artillery, circa 1934. BELOW As sergeant, artillery, circa 1937.

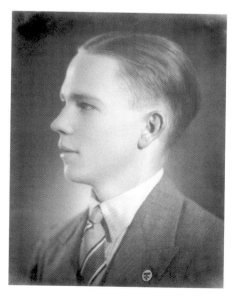

LEFT In 1939 I graduated from the University of Sydney with MB BS.

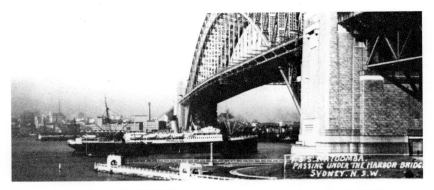

COURTESY OF THE LATE MRS FLORENCE O'NEILL

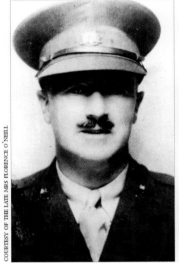

ABOVE Embarkation day, July 1941. We set sail from Sydney on the *Katoomba*, bound for Perth.

ABOVE Our much-loved Commanding Officer 2/15th Field Regiment AIF, Lieutenant Colonel John O'Neill. His accidental death in November 1941 in Malaya was devastating for all of his men.

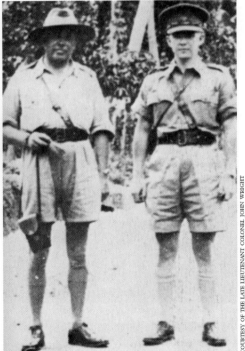

COURTESY OF THE LATE LIEUTENANT COLONEL JOHN WRIGHT

ABOVE The new Commanding Officer 2/15th Field Regiment AIF, Lieutenant Colonel John Wright (left) with me. Here we were on leave from Tampin in 1941.

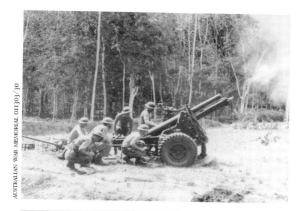

LEFT Men of the 2/15th Field Regiment firing a British-made 25-pounder gun from a clearing near Bakri in 1942.

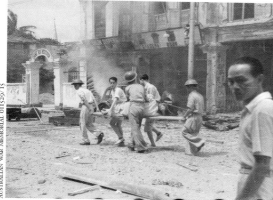

LEFT The defence of the supposedly 'impregnable' Singapore Island was a myth. During February 1942, wounded men were carried on stretchers to casualty clearing stations while bombs fell.

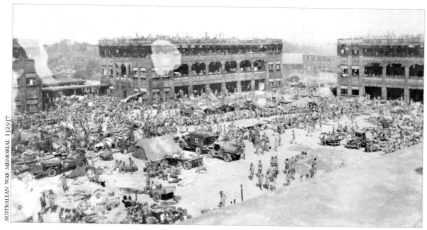

ABOVE AIF and British troops flooding into Selerang Barracks, Changi, Singapore, 9 February 1942. I arrived at Birdwood Camp, a satellite camp located within the Changi area, nine days later.

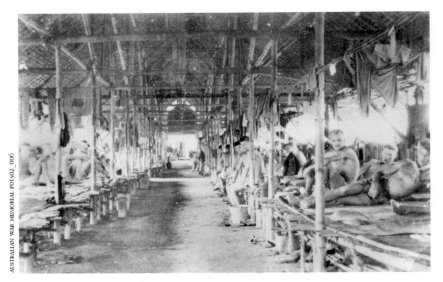

ABOVE A bamboo and *attap* hut, typical of some of the better accommodation in fixed camps. The huts housing us in Railway construction camps were of the same design but much more decrepit and filthy.

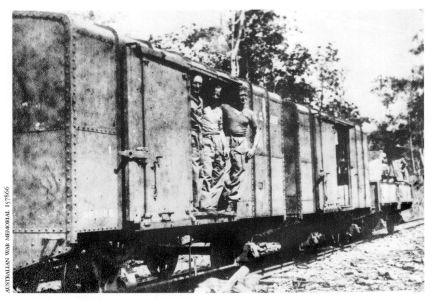

ABOVE Enclosed steel wagons typical of those used to transport prisoners of war. Each wagon featured a single sliding door in the centre, and most men jostled for a position near the opening. Men were packed in tightly, up to 40 men per wagon, in unbearably hot conditions.

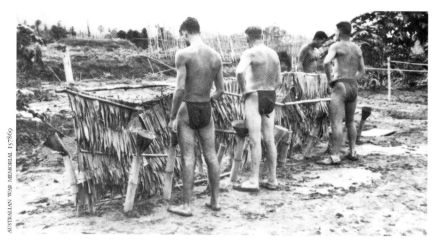

ABOVE Prisoners of war dressed in G-strings, often the only item of clothing they still had in their possession. This urinal is typical of those built by the men in Railway camps, also known as 'pissophones' by the men.

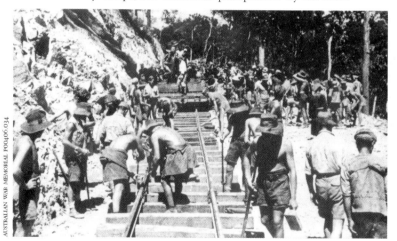

ABOVE Australian and British prisoners of war, members of 'A' Force, laying track on the Railway. Line laying was extremely strenuous work for sick and malnourished men.

RIGHT Improvisation was essential for survival as a prisoner of war. The men made their own clogs from teak and canvas.

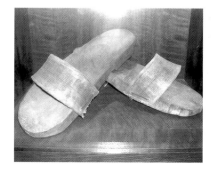

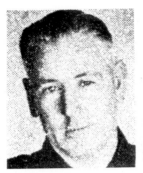

LEFT Jim Armstrong, known as 'Old Silver', my medical orderly and friend. He was a tireless and dedicated orderly who never gave up. He saved the lives of many men.

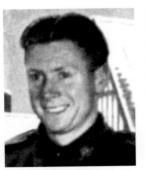

LEFT Pinkey Rhodes, another dedicated medical orderly and friend. He is the sole remaining medical orderly from my group.

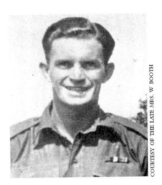

ABOVE Don Booth, another medical orderly and friend. Don was also our Regimental bugler.

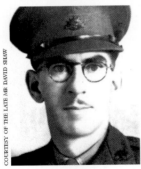

LEFT My closest friend and confidant along the Railway, John Shaw. John had a profound effect on my life both as a prisoner of war and in the years that followed.

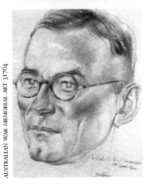

LEFT Commander of Anderson Force in Burma and Thailand, Lieutenant Colonel Charles Anderson, VC, MC. He maintained a high level of morale among his men.

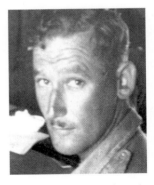

ABOVE My lifelong friend Des Makepeace. This photograph was taken in 1941 in Tampin, Malaya.

A clear system of hierarchy quickly became apparent. Within the Japanese Army, it seemed every Japanese soldier was entitled to bash a fellow Japanese soldier of a lower rank: colonels bashed majors, majors bashed captains and so it continued down the line. We witnessed this first-hand on a regular basis. All Japanese were then entitled to bash Koreans of any rank. We, of course, sat at the very bottom of this pecking order, copping it from both directions, and before long I was on the receiving end of a thrashing from Peanut.

One morning Peanut approached me in the RAP and demanded that I order extra men from camp to go out to work on the Railway. We had already supplied our required quota of men for the day but the Japanese engineers had sent word back to Peanut that they wanted even more men. I calmly told Peanut that all men in camp were too sick to work. 'Byoki [sick]. Malaria. Beriberi. Dysentery,' I said, shaking my head.

Peanut's forehead creased in rage; his eyes seemed even closer together when he was angry. 'Shigoto! [work],' he yelled. 'Shigoto!'

I shook my head again. 'No.'

Peanut lunged at me with his bamboo stick, beating me about the head and shoulders. His arms flapped in a fury. The bamboo whistled through the air in between each strike. I tried not to flinch — I didn't want to give him the satisfaction of seeing any sign of the pain he was inflicting. A prisoner of war's only defence while being beaten was to keep his eyes wide open, so you could see the punches coming and 'roll with them' as best you could (after the war, I learned that the Japanese considered it the ultimate in disrespect to stare at them during punishment, but I was unaware of this at the time). More than anything I was worried about my specs. I was dependent on them to do my job properly. I had a spare pair in my pack, but who knew when they might be confiscated and ground underfoot by a guard — a common act of bastardy. I don't recall how long my punishment lasted; time, it seemed, stood still during a beating. When the whipping finally stopped, I looked up at Peanut through my thankfully unscathed glasses. His face was lobster red. I pointed towards our own camp headquarters, indicating that he would need to speak to Captain Drower or Colonel Anderson if he wanted to take matters further. Peanut swivelled on the heels of his boots and stamped out of the RAP, leaving my sick men in their beds and me with bloodied but not serious lacerations and contusions to my head, neck and face. He had caused more damage to my ego than my skin, but the attack was an early warning of what Peanut was capable of dealing out to prisoners.

AT THE END OF the month we received our first pay since leaving Tavoy. After the standard deductions for our Red Cross fund and for 'board and lodging' by the Japanese, I was left with twenty rupees to spend in the canteen or give to those men who were in desperate need of additional food. Black market activity continued to boom: men traded with the Burmese as well as Japanese and Korean guards. Watches, fountain pens and cigarette lighters were highly prized items; most men only had one of each, so they rapidly ran out of treasures to trade.

With the year almost over, we prepared to celebrate our first Christmas in captivity in a truly festive manner. Extra titbits were purchased from the Burmese traders using profits from our canteen to stockpile food for a rare feast.[3] The men also took responsibility for tasks such as wrapping 'presents' and decorating a tree. The Japanese declared Christmas Day would be a day of rest, but that was as far as their generosity stretched.

In the early hours of Christmas morning I was woken by a guard and ordered to see another Japanese guard who was suffering a bellyache. The Japanese had their own medical orderlies in the camps, but their doctors were located at headquarters at Thanbyuzayat, so they didn't hesitate to call on me on this occasion. The guard was suffering the consequences of gorging on green bananas. Gluttony was my silent diagnosis. Without sympathy, I gave him a couple of well-known 'Number 9' army tablets — a violent laxative reputedly capable of moving mountains. Aside from causing a fair amount of discomfort, the tablets were harmless and, like my men, I wasn't above claiming petty victories when the opportunity arose.

By the time I left my grateful and oblivious patient, dawn was glowing, so rather than return to bed I called on Jim Armstrong; I wanted to be the first to wish him a Merry Christmas. In hand was the hipflask I had filled with brandy before leaving Changi; I'd been saving it for a special occasion. Jim and I shared a small tot together and were soon joined by Bob Kemp, a medical orderly from the engineers. We three enjoyed what amounted to a sip in total, but we savoured it as a genuine indulgence.

I held a very brief sick parade in the morning before our celebrations in camp commenced in earnest. Members of the 22nd Brigade band, most of whom were with Ramsay Force and had somehow managed to retain their instruments, paid us a visit before lunch. They entertained us with a delightful musical line-up, including: 'Waltzing Matilda', followed by a Japanese number; Christmas carols 'Come All Ye Faithful' and 'Christians Awake'; 'Pack Up Your Troubles'; 'The Sharp Shooter'; 'The Georgian Camp Meeting'; 'The Flying Eagle'; 'Wings Over the Navy'; 'Colonel Bogey'; and finally 'Auld Lang Syne'. It was the first music we had heard for months, apart from the tuneless Japanese flutes some of the guards played from time to time.

Our lads put on their own concert after tea, complete with a real live Father Christmas played by one of our sergeants, 'Slapdash' Purdy, with padded belly and a white beard and cap made from God only knows what. Every sergeant was presented with a small parcel containing an article that had been secretly removed from the innermost recesses of his kit bag by 'Santa's little helpers'. Men unwrapped their parcels only to discover a pair of their own socks, a cigarette case or some other personal treasure. They were delighted all the same.

Some of the men made tasty puddings over campfires from hand-ground rice flour, *chindegar*, eggs, and dripping. The dripping came from suet our men discreetly snatched from various beasts the Japanese had ordered them to slaughter (to provide food for the guards, of course, not us). Not a hungry man could be found in camp that night. After each meal of the day, Syd Krantz (a surgeon with the casualty clearing station), Don Murchison (our International Red Cross representative) and I enjoyed a real cigarette — a Players — which they had been carrying in their tin containers. I also smoked a pipe of Ranch tobacco I'd been saving from a parcel I received from home last Christmas during action. I delighted in every puff.

Merriment prevailed all day, but when the sun went down, I felt enormously homesick. My thoughts were very much with my mother and father in Sydney, and family in Kyogle, where I had spent so many Christmases before the war. I thought of Uncle Arthur, who always insisted on what he called a 'postprandial conference' (a sleep) after Christmas lunch, and tried to imagine what they were all doing this year. Before going to bed, I wrote in my diary — a new diary. My first notebook was now full, so I wrapped it carefully in a sheet of paper and concealed it in the bottom of my pack. I commenced my second diary in a fresh notebook, recording the wonderful events of the day and listing specific details of the three meals we had relished. Emotionally exhausted and nostalgic, I went to sleep wondering how many more pages I would have to fill before we made it home again.

ON BOXING DAY OUR festivities ended with a chilling discovery: the bloodied body of one of our men, Sergeant Ronnie O'Donnell. When O'Donnell failed to appear at roll call, the men had conducted their own search and soon found his body in the jungle, not far from where they had been working. He had been shot by Peanut Tomoto, the same guard who had bashed me not so long ago.

Peanut claimed O'Donnell was attempting escape when he shot him, despite the fact O'Donnell had been killed by a bullet through the front of his chest (two more shots had also been fired through his head whilst he was lying down, presumably after death). It was sheer murder: committed, we believed, through panic or temporary insanity. Some speculated that Peanut may have been seeking retribution for O'Donnell rejecting sexual advances, but none of us will ever know the truth.

We were outraged, and some of the men were nearing breaking point. Fearing unrest and retaliation from us, the Japanese whisked Peanut off to Thanbyuzayat, promising further investigation into the matter by Nagatomo at Japanese Headquarters. The Japanese refused to allow me to view O'Donnell's body before sending it to Thanbyuzayat for burial.

Nagatomo's findings condoned Peanut's actions: he agreed the Korean guard had simply been carrying out Japanese orders to shoot any man 'attempting escape'. We expected as much. When Peanut was returned to duty some time later, we renamed him 'Dillinger', after the notorious 1930s American criminal, John Dillinger.

The death of O'Donnell was further confirmation that our lives no longer belonged to us. To the Japanese, the life of a prisoner of war was worthless; we were totally expendable. O'Donnell's murder left the rest of us with a sense of powerlessness and the understanding that more deaths would follow. Lives could be lost in an instant — erased — with no opportunity for justice or retaliation.

IN CAPTIVITY, TO HAVE mates you had to be a mate. I never saw an Australian who did not have some one to care for him when ill, in times of hardship or to simply raise his spirits. Over the past few months I had been forging a strong new friendship with Major John Shaw. In addition to being an engineer, John had worked as a builder with his father, a master builder, and had studied architecture; he also possessed a profound knowledge of literature, music and philosophy. John never talked down or up to anybody. He could discuss the arts with professors in the same way he spoke to a labourer about how to dig a drain with a pick and shovel. He respected all men equally.

A former cyclist, John was a tall and distinguished-looking man with solid legs that in days to come would waste away to loose skin on bone. He introduced me to the wide world of literature and philosophy through regular one-on-one lectures and, above all else, he helped me to think in new ways. I was then 26 years old and John was fourteen years my senior. He was a wise owl and I was his pupil. Extremely tolerant of my ignorance (me, the former schoolboy who had questioned intended meanings in the works of Shakespeare!), and unfailingly patient, he never made me feel the fool I was. John Shaw became my confidant, mentor and closest friend.

Together we spent a great deal of time contemplating what we would do 'after the war': it never occurred to either of us that Allied forces would not win, or that we might not return home. Once the United States entered the war, our optimism had increased and we had been hearing word-of-mouth reports about recent Allied successes, including the recapture of Kokoda by Australian troops, Rommel's defeat in El Alamein and Allied victory at Guadalcanal (British Solomon Islands). I sought John's advice as to whether I should establish a general practice in the city or the country and we discussed the merits of both. I nominated Kyogle, Newcastle and Taree as my preferred country destinations, and Seaforth and Cronulla as my Sydney options. John helped me narrow my choice to Kyogle or Seaforth. After hours of discussion, I decided on Seaforth, where I could apply for residency at Manly Hospital before joining a medical group practice; at the same time, I could maintain my contacts with the Mater Hospital in North Sydney. I immediately began drawing plans for a house suitable for my harbourside location (featuring a sun porch, a large hallway, and a lobby with a separate medical wing!). Excited, my mind whirring with ideas and thoughts of settling at Seaforth, I was unable to sleep properly for the next few nights, including New Year's Eve.

On New Year's Day I woke filled with hope. Over the past few days John Shaw had set my mind alight with renewed inspiration, keeping me focused on a much brighter future. Looking back I realise my ongoing discussions with John undoubtedly ensured I would never degenerate into leading an animal or vegetable existence: he had a profound effect on my life both as a prisoner of war and in the years that followed.

The Japanese granted us a day of rest to welcome the New Year and once again, our cooks excelled themselves. We enjoyed a special pudding, complete with brandy sauce, a real treat, followed by a sleep and bridge in the afternoon. I celebrated Hogmanay with Jim and the rest of my RAP staff in the right spirit with yet another tot of precious brandy. I hoped like hell that 1943 would be the year of our liberation — I had so much now to look forward to.

CHAPTER EIGHT

A NEW YEAR
Hlepauk (18 Kilo camp) to Tan Yin (35 Kilo camp)
January–March 1943

The first of twenty trucks arrived just before lunchtime on 3 January to transport us to our next camp, Tan Yin (35 Kilo camp). Before departing, I received a rare and unexplained 'gift' of medical supplies courtesy of the Japanese: two dozen bandages, six metres of lint, 30 grams of potassium permanganate, 60 grams of aspirin, 120 grams of magnesium sulphate and two small tins of throat pastilles. While grossly inadequate for a camp strength numbering 600, it was extravagant in comparison to previous supplies.

Tan Yin was in a far better state than Hlepauk. Members of Williams Force had been here for several weeks already, and had successfully established a high standard of hygiene and sanitation. Made up chiefly of the 2/2nd Pioneer Battalion under the command of Lieutenant Colonel John Williams, Williams Force had been sailing in convoy from the Middle East, towards Singapore, when they were diverted to Java. After a short, sharp scrap they found themselves prisoners of the Japanese. Colonel

Williams, among others, spent six weeks in the 'bicycle investigation camp' where to obtain information the Japanese had forced bamboo slivers beneath the fingernails of prisoners (along with other not-so-gentle encouragements). Also amongst those of Williams Force were survivors of HMAS *Perth*, which was sunk off the coast of Java in the Sunda Strait on 28 February 1942.

Our new camp featured a glorious view of hills, including one with a large and magnificent bluff. Burma was beautiful; I never tired of the trees and the hills, or the ever-changing effects of sun and shade. Our huts, made of the usual bamboo with *attap* roofs, featured a raised platform approximately four metres wide and 100 metres long, divided into bays. By jungle standards, they were well built. The biggest disadvantage of our new location was that there was no river. Water had to be drawn from wells using a 'whip' — a long bamboo pole weighted at one end and with a bucket dangling from the other.

In cooperation with Williams Force, further camp construction was soon in progress. Lieutenant Colonel Norman Eadie, the medical officer attached to Williams Force, had already established a serviceable hospital and RAP: he opened his kit on the bamboo sleeping deck for the duration of his sick parade, then packed it away again. The Japanese promised we would receive a tent we could use as a combined RAP and hospital, but I wasn't holding my breath.

Our men were forced to work even longer hours on the Railway embankment. Each day they had to collect archaic tools and equipment from the storehouse at camp and carry them to and from their worksite, where their now bony bodies were expected to labour from dawn until 1900 hours, with only miserably short meal and rest breaks in between. They were expected to achieve 1.4 to 1.6 cubic metres of excavation of red-clay soil per man per day, in addition to coping with a seven-kilometre return journey on foot.

The Japanese also began increasing their daily quota of men required to work. In response, we developed a carefully calculated system to conserve our 'manpower'. During the morning sick parade, along with Jim Armstrong and the medical orderlies, Allan Taylor, a clerical sergeant, meticulously recorded the medical history of each man. A former bank manager, Allan had a mind like a steel trap: without even looking at his records he could tell me how many attacks of malaria a particular man had endured, the date of his last attack of dysentery and any other medical detail of importance. Also ever present was 2 i/c of Anderson Force, Major Don Kerr, who faithfully kept the sick parade roll and noted the classification of each man ('Duty'; 'Light Duty'; 'No Duty'; or 'Hospital'). After dark, when the workers returned to camp, I held yet another sick parade for those who had become ill on the job, with Don Kerr again carefully noting the classification of each man. Don and I then spent hours each night working our way through the roll together, reviewing every man on paper. Any man who had been at work for more than seven to ten consecutive days, we automatically marked 'No Duty' for the next day and 'Duty' for the following day.

We became adept at forecasting the number of men the Japanese would demand to work each day and, with an estimated figure in mind, we counted how many we had marked 'Duty'. If we were short on numbers, some who had been marked 'Light Duty' or 'No Duty' would have to go to work. We would review these cases again to establish which men would suffer the least harm by being sent to work. It was not a matter of determining if a man was unfit or fit, but rather evaluating the relative unfitness of one man against another. Each night we circulated our lists in advance to the men, and never once did I hear of a complaint from the sick who had to work in order that the not-so-sick could have one rest day in camp. Manipulating these figures took a lot of time, but we were convinced there would be long-term benefit: prevention in the form of rest was one of the few medicines we could prescribe.

As my Japanese language skills improved, so too did my results in bargaining with the guards. The Japanese frequently initiated 'blitz' sick parades, during which one of their guards — medically unqualified — was ordered to scrutinise our sick men. Such inspections quickly turned into human auctions when, at times, prudent bidding could mean the difference between life and death. With the men ordered on parade, accompanied by a guard, I moved down the line. Haggling commenced with my initial offer.

'This man, Malaria. No duty, five days.'

Invariably the guard by my side would disagree: 'No. One day.'

I would shake my head. 'No. Very sick. Four days,' holding up four fingers.

If I was lucky, the guard would come back with another counter offer: 'Two days.'

Then quickly I would offer 'three days', with three fingers held in the air.

Bang. Sold! The first deal of the day was done and bargaining continued, one man at a time. At all times I had to be careful not to push the guard too far. If he insisted on sending a sick man to work, one whom I knew would come to no great harm as a result, I did not contest unduly. However, when we came to a man who was dangerously ill, I argued vigorously and usually managed to gain a reprieve, even if only for a day. Generally, guards were more willing to negotiate over men suffering from conditions where outward signs were displayed, such as tropical ulcers or oedema from 'wet' beriberi, than they were in regard to more serious conditions, such as pellagra or 'dry' beriberi, where there were very few obvious physical symptoms.

Reflecting now on my role as RMO, the level of responsibility I was given appals me. I was playing God, deciding who would go to work, who would receive an extra egg or spoonful of rice, who was allowed a day of rest in camp. Surely I should have experienced some remorse, but at the time I cannot remember regretting a single decision I made. Whether this was a matter of denial — that I pushed any guilt out of my mind so I could keep going — I don't know. Maybe. But when I was reviewing hundreds of men on parade at a time, I didn't have long to make up my mind. I didn't have the luxury of going back and saying, 'Gee, wish I hadn't done that.' I had to make a split-second decision, the best decision I could, and move on to the next man in line.

I WAS PLEASANTLY SURPRISED when the Japanese gave me three six-metre tents to be used for medical facilities, to be followed by the delivery of floorboards. We pitched the tents, pleased to be at least close to establishing an RAP and hospital. The number of sick was fairly steady at 200, including about 30 'chronic unfits' who had recently returned from the base hospital at Thanbyuzayat. When the sick travelled to and from Thanbyuzayat they always brought news, sometimes even letters from friends in other camps, as well as whatever food they could buy and carry. The Japanese used prisoners of war to drive the ration trucks to and from headquarters, and our economic officers were also required to travel back to Thanbyuzayat on a regular basis to collect the pay. The value of these 'carrier pigeons' was immeasurable.

Word soon reached us that Nagatomo had returned to Thanbyuzayat from Singapore (where he had been briefly summoned) and was apparently a reformed character. He was said to have purchased large quantities of sporting gear and built two tennis courts at headquarters. Furthermore, football fields were soon to be built in each camp and a Red Cross ship was on its way. And pigs might fly, too.

While the men on the Railway endured unremitting heat during the day, trudging off to work often in no more than a G-string, the nights were bitterly cold. A small number of men still had a groundsheet or blanket, but many had long ago traded theirs for food. The only way to keep warm was to don every item of clothing we possessed, which wasn't much. Three weeks into our stay at this new camp, there was a surge in URTIs (upper respiratory tract infections) — coughs, cold and flu, and early stages of pellagra, mainly in the form of inflammation and painful swelling of the tongue. More than 300 men were now reporting daily on sick parade, including 60 with URTIs and 120 with early stages of pellagra. I feared we were heading for a pellagra epidemic.

I was beginning to notice that the big, bronzed Aussie blokes and the younger men weren't faring so well as others. Considering a man who was formerly 60 or 65 kilograms received the same pitiful rations as one who was 90 kilograms, it was hardly surprising the larger blokes faced a greater struggle, while the youngest men probably suffered more because of their limited military experience. I liken it to a comparison between a young bull and an old bull. Imagine a young bull and an old bull travelling over the crest of a hill and looking down with pleasurable anticipation at some attractive heifers below. The young bull says, 'Let's dash down and grab a couple,' and the old bull says, 'Let's go quietly and get the lot.' Likewise, the more mature of our blokes were far better at pacing themselves — at work, with their rations and with their expectations. They also had a heightened sense of mortality.

By the end of January, the number on sick parade reached a massive 412, and many of the pellagra cases progressed from the first stage of dermatitis to the second stage of diarrhoea: I feared that dementia and death would soon follow for some. With so many sick men in camp, the Japanese ordered one four-grain tablet of quinine be given to each man on evening *tenko*. Such a quantity was useless for the suppression of malaria, and only served in depleting valuable supplies which could have been used for treatment. According to their logic, if the men were given suppressive quinine there would be no malaria and, therefore, no need for any further supplies for treatment to be issued. It was a waste of time trying to understand how they ever came to such a conclusion — or indeed why they were focusing on malaria in the midst of a pellagra outbreak.

We issued all men 45 to 60 grams of *chindegar* yeast per day, with an extra 30 or 60 grams for those suffering from pellagra. The Japanese refused to allow us to establish our own canteen at this camp, so with little to work with other than rice, the cooks did an excellent job of producing an array of bread and biscuits. The bread was made by mixing a dough of rice flour, ground by placing the rice between two horizontally revolving stones, and leavened with our homemade yeast. This dough, after standing, was baked in ovens made from cut-down 44-gallon oil drums covered with mud. Primitive, but effective. The biscuits were made from the coarser ground rice, which was rolled into a pastry and baked. With a slightly better diet containing much needed yeast, the pellagra position finally started to improve by early February. Our homemade yeast was proving to be more effective than I initially suspected,[1] with sick figures starting to drop at the rate of about ten men a day. While those with pellagra in its early stages showed signs of recovery the more advanced cases remained a concern, especially those with diarrhoea. I had further arguments with the Japanese over sending the sick to work and we eventually reached an agreement whereby very sick men would only work on alternate days, and only had to achieve 0.8 cubic metres of excavation a day — half the current required work rate. Small but important concessions for ill men.

BRIGADIER VARLEY AND Major Ted Fisher (who was then in charge of the base hospital at Thanbyuzayat) visited our camp on 10 February in company with Nagatomo and Lieutenant Dr

Higuchi, a Japanese doctor. Ted Fisher inspected the pellagra cases and agreed entirely with my diagnosis and opinions. Following the inspection, the visitors and local commanders held a conference at which it was agreed that meat and other foods would be purchased locally for the men. Salvation at last, I thought.

Despite the support I received from Major Fisher, Colonel Anderson, our commanding officer, questioned the seriousness of the medical condition of our troops, particularly in regard to pellagra, a disease he failed to understand. Unspoken tension between Anderson and me had been building for weeks now, and it was about to surface.

Anderson was 46 years old and a big man both in stature and by reputation. He wore large, horn-rimmed glasses that seemed to magnify his eyes. A distinctive dimple pocked his chin. Born in South Africa, Anderson was awarded a Military Cross in the First World War — fighting in the jungles of East Africa with the King's African Rifles — and then spent time as a big-game hunter in the jungles of Kenya. His jungle experience had proved invaluable in the Malayan campaign, where his fearless and inspired leadership in the epic battle of Muar earned him the Victoria Cross and the undying respect and admiration of the men not only of his 2/19th Battalion, but also of 'A' Force, all of whom would have followed him to hell and back.

I was becoming increasingly frustrated that Colonel Anderson did not appear to be willing to stand up to the Japanese by refusing to allow sick men to work. I had been working non-stop for weeks on end, barely sleeping and suffering from an URTI. I needed his support. Anderson, no doubt influenced by his experience as a big-game hunter in Africa, took a 'softly softly catchee monkey' approach with our keepers. He believed it was better not to antagonise them, but rather go along with them, diplomatically educating them about the needs of our men. When his sweet talking failed he passed the Japanese on to me or recommended that our keepers run their own sick parade, with inevitable, disastrous results.

Anderson's approach was very different from that of Colonel Williams, commanding officer of Williams Force. Both Anderson and Williams possessed impeccable military records for courage, bravery, leadership and command in action, and neither demanded nor expected special privileges usually accorded to commanding officers, but Williams, having been personally tortured by the Japanese, and undoubtedly influenced by his own engineering and Pioneer experience, chose to deal with our keepers head on. He disagreed and argued with guards, often at great personal expense in the form of beatings. History records that there was merit in both of the very different tactics employed by each in dealing with the Japanese, and it is a moot point which colonel caused more or less trouble for his men as a result but, at the time, I was far more in favour of Colonel Williams' approach.

Anderson and I reached our first major breaking point when he insisted on sending sick men to work on the Railway against my advice. I respected him greatly for his heroic service record, and obviously he was a colonel and I was a captain, but I stated my case for the men not working in a way that let him know how I really felt. (Looking back, I can see that the way I stated my case probably didn't help matters between us.) Clearly, as our commanding officer, Anderson was charged with ultimate responsibility for his men — but he was not medically trained and, on medical matters, it was normal to accept the advice of one with medical training. He maintained that 'opinions' should always be queried and not necessarily accepted, which I couldn't dispute, but to me it was more a question of whether he was seeking clarification or ignoring my advice. I suspected the latter.

Behind closed doors, Anderson accused me of being off-handed and claimed I had no bedside manner. 'The men have no confidence in you,' he said. These are words I will never forget. My face went blank. I was stunned. His accusations were personally devastating — and bewildering. I denied them vehemently.

Colonel Anderson summoned Major Kerr, who knew nothing of my troubles with Anderson, and asked him if he believed I had the confidence and respect of the troops. Major Kerr, standing in front of both Anderson and me, looked puzzled.

'Of course he does,' Kerr said. I didn't know where to look. Anderson continued his line of questioning and Kerr continued to offer his support for me. It was humiliating: the last thing I wanted was for our commanding officer, who was so highly revered by his men, to be seen to be unsupportive of his RMO. Anderson apparently accepted Kerr's responses as the truth, but offered no apology or explanation for his unfounded allegations. Shattered by his lack of confidence in me, I requested to be transferred to another unit. Anderson refused, signalling what I hoped might be a truce — and the beginning of a more harmonious relationship between us in days to come.

THE NIGHTS BECAME WARMER during February. Every evening there was a glorious sunset, the predominant colours of pink and rose were reflected on the mountains. The sick figures dropped a little further and the Japanese promptly suspended the initiative of sick men only working alternate days. Our meat ration was increased to 150 grams, but only on paper, in reality it rarely exceeded 50 grams. We continued to hammer our keepers for canteen facilities but without success. One saving grace was that the Japanese were now allowing me to send some men to Thanbyuzayat to receive dental treatment. Any dental work was of secondary consideration; a trip to headquarters meant another opportunity for the men to sneak back into camp rare delicacies such as tomatoes, onions, peanuts, and even peanut toffee.

The fifteenth of February marked our first anniversary of becoming prisoners of war. To celebrate, we heard that Nagatomo ordered a soccer match of prisoners of war versus the Japanese at Thanbyuzayat. Our spirits lifted when we learned that our team defeated them 3–1 (with the prisoners of war being ordered to take it easy in the second half). The following night the Japanese held a big party at our own camp to farewell a popular Japanese lieutenant, Yamada, and welcome his replacement, Lieutenant Asoto. They demanded our 'orchestra'[2] play and sing the Japanese version of 'They'll be Dropping Thousand Pounders When They Come'. In place of 'Ai Ai Yippy Yippy Ai' our men sang 'Ni Ni Nippy Nippy Ni'. *Ni* means 'no' in Japanese, so we enjoyed hearing the Japanese singing along to their own swan song, completely oblivious to our joke.

Asoto appeared to be quite a decent guard: initially he was not actively aggressive and he seemed to profess sympathy for the sick. One night I was suturing a small wound on a lad's hand when Asoto arrived on the scene to inspect our hospital. He found the sight of the bloody wound so upsetting he left immediately. Only half an hour later I heard some terrific screams coming from the direction of the guardhouse. Asoto was in the process of bashing one of his guards into a messy pulp — breaking the guard's ribs in the process.

EARLY ON 1 MARCH, at 0220 hours, Thanbyuzayat experienced its first big bombing raid. Some damage, extent unknown, was done in a rubber plantation about two kilometres along the Moulmein line. It was a stark reminder that the war was still happening around us, and yet another opportunity for us to optimistically believe that the Brits or Yanks might be on their way to rescue us. We had been keeping up to date with such events, as well as the progress of the war, thanks to the operation of an improvised and illicit camp radio. Nowhere in my diary did I make a single mention, even by implication, of news events: the penalty for having a radio would have been death. Initially assembled in Tavoy from 'acquired' parts — valves, wires and batteries — the radio was manned by two engineers, Lieutenant Arthur Watchorn and Sergeant Roy Wilstencroft, who mainly listened to the BBC. They passed world news on to Colonel Anderson, who mostly passed on to us what we suspected were sanitised versions of events. We had to be very careful that the guards didn't hear us discussing news of the war. For some, this was no easy task. One of our sergeants, Tommy Smith, was renowned for continually putting his foot in it; he was the type of bloke who couldn't see a tree if he was walking into it. On one occasion he bolted up to a group of us and, in front of a guard, excitedly announced a fresh piece of news about Allied forces. Remarkably, the sleepy guard didn't twig, and one of our quick-thinking men grabbed Tommy and hustled him around the corner of a hut, but it was a close call. Whenever we moved camps, the radio was sewn inside a bag of rice from the Japanese kitchen, which the Japanese unknowingly transported for us!

Our rations in camp remained NBG (no bloody good); for days at a time we received no meat at all. Hunger had become an accepted part of our life. I considered myself lucky to have grown up during the Great Depression. If I had remained the pudgy schoolboy I used to be, my struggle now would have been even greater. Early on in captivity, back in Tavoy, eating had been a complete obsession for some — many of the men had passed time trading recipes with the Dutch and planning what they would eat when they returned home — but by now food was just like sex, we tried not to think about it.

Towards the end of the month we received a sudden order to move all our sick to the newly established 30 Kilo hospital camp at Retpu. All men we had marked as 'No Duty' for that day, some of whom were still relatively fit and just enjoying an unofficial day of rest, were evacuated to the hospital, along with Colonel Eadie (the medical officer attached to Williams Force) and surgeon Syd Krantz. With increasing *speedo! speedo!* pressure on the Railway, the Japanese now reasoned that if all the sick were in hospital, all those who remained would be fit from here on in.

It seemed likely the rest of us would be moving to the 26 Kilo camp, at Kunknitkway, but plans changed daily. Individual work parties were allocated different tasks to perform, whether it was embankment work, line laying, bridge building or anything else the Japanese ordered. If there was an emergency, such as a bridge being washed away, or urgent repair works required, the Japanese could suddenly order a group to move to a new location to fix the problem. We never knew where we were headed next, nor did we care. A man could make himself sick from speculation and besides, wherever we were sent, we would still be on the Railway and under the rule of the Japanese.

CHAPTER NINE

LINE LAYING
Tan Yin (35 Kilo camp) to Kunknitkway (26 Kilo camp)
March–April 1943

Very early on the morning of 8 March, we set off north on yet
another journey on foot. With other groups of POWs already
situated at camps further south to continue road building,
embankment and bridge work, our men now faced the task of
line laying on the already completed embankments, starting at
Kunknitkway (26 Kilo camp) and working their way south.
Anderson Force had, by this stage, been officially combined with
Williams Force, to be known as the No. 1 Mobile Force.

We marched under the cover of darkness. The sky seemed to
lower, laden with bruised clouds, and we were soon saturated by
the first heavy shower of rain we had experienced since the wet
season. The rain was warm but showed no sign of easing up. We
struggled to stay on our feet, slipping on the red clay soil of the
Railway embankment with guards screeching at us to keep pace.
Forced to keep in close contact to maintain our balance, we each
rested one hand on the pack of the man in front of us: we formed
a long line of bony frames linked like a daisy chain. When it came

to crossing the bridges, there were neither sleepers nor rails, just two parallel timbers about twenty centimetres wide, on which we had to balance barefooted and burdened with heavy packs, inching our way across. How no one tumbled off a bridge, one of which was more than 30 metres above a river bed, I cannot say. It was so dark (the black of night and early morning in the jungle is the darkest black you can imagine); perhaps the fact that we couldn't see stopped us from becoming dizzy and overbalancing. Some would, no doubt, give credit to the Almighty.

Completely buggered, our bodies crying out for rest and food, we arrived at Kunknitkway just before dawn to find a BA (bloody awful) camp: it was to be our new home. There were flies and filth everywhere, hopelessly inadequate huts with not enough room to accommodate all of us, and rain leaking through the *attap* walls and roofs. The foul stench of yak faeces was overwhelming — dung of the devil. The place was a miserable dump.

During our last four days at Tan Yin, we hadn't received any rations. Now the guards were pointing to maggot-infested mounds in front of us, informing us that they had delivered our rations here instead. We were sickened by the waste of such desperately needed food. I looked around me — the faces of men were sallow, their eyes sunken and their ribs starting to jut through thin skin. The physical transition from burly soldiers to slaves surviving on a starvation diet had been gradual over the past months, and most men had already become accustomed to each other's skeletal form.

In the tropics, the dense undergrowth grows very quickly, collecting rubbish and filth in the process and creating a fertile breeding ground for flies. The state of this camp was of grave concern: severe diarrhoea would be inevitable, at the very least. Cleaning and clearing the place without supplies was a difficult, almost futile task, and with the men ordered to work long days on the Railway, the only help I had access to was from the sick. None of us was ready to admit defeat — after all, we were surviving —

but I couldn't help wondering how long it would be before men started to drop dead around me. The combination of heavy line-laying work on top of malnutrition and inadequate medical supplies would surely prove a lethal mix. If this camp was any indication of what lay ahead, even those with the toughest determination would need bags of luck to make it through.

DURING OUR SECOND MORNING at Kunknitkway, a Japanese truck lurched into camp. Great excitement ensued when Lieutenant Naito, lying inert and bloody on a wire mattress, was unloaded and carried towards his billet. Naito was already well known to us: he had been temporarily in charge of our group when Nagatomo was called to Singapore. We had experienced little face-to-face contact with him up until now, but his reputation as a brutal drunk preceded him. Also well known was the obvious tension between Naito and his superior. According to rumours between the camps, Nagatomo frequently bashed Naito, and looking at Naito's battered body in front of us, now I believed it. Word quickly spread that Naito had been repeatedly kicked by Nagatomo following yet another disagreement between the loveless pair. Naito, covered in cuts and bruises and moaning in pain, called for 'the boy doctor'.[1]

Inside the billet, Naito was grunting like an injured pig. 'Help,' he slurred, pointing to his cuts and bruises.

I could smell alcohol on his breath. He was drunk, the corners of his mouth wet with drool creeping its way down his chin. He greeted me with a grim smile, seemingly grateful to have me by his side. Older than his fellow Japanese officers and nearly all of the guards, Naito was less able to cope with pain than most. He was physically softer, reportedly a banker prior to his army days, and not the usual army type.

Back then, the medical profession believed that heat applied to abrasions in the form of hot foments would increase blood circulation and promote healing, and massage was considered an effective treatment for bruising. I borrowed sweat towels (similar to a barber's towel) from some of the guards, who often wore them around their necks during the day. I boiled the little towels in water before placing them on Naito's cuts and then vigorously massaged his bruises. Lying back on the mattress like an obedient child, Naito groaned while I worked on him but he didn't abuse or threaten me; he seemed to relish the attention. (The treatment was painful but it was also the accepted practice at the time — although I would be lying if I didn't admit that I was quietly hoping the cure might prove to be even more agonising than his complaints.) After I removed the foments and got up to leave, Naito declared: 'You very clever doctor.' Looking down at the floorboards, I rubbed the back of my neck with one hand before raising my head to offer a bland smile in return: I couldn't care less what a man like Naito thought of me.

THE DAYS WERE STILL very hot and storm clouds continued to arrive, lashing rain soaking the soil. The wet season was upon us — again — and with it came renewed concern about dysentery and diarrhoea, as well as the risk of cholera. The camp grounds would soon be a muddy quagmire.

While I attended to the sick in camp, out on the Railway, men were ordered to unload heavy teak sleepers from rail bogies and lay them in position. Spiking gangs drilled holes in the sleepers with hand augers — a tool resembling a corkscrew — ready to be 'spiked'. The spikers then had to drive steel rail spikes into the holes with poor quality four-kilogram hammers; fragments of steel became flying pieces of shrapnel which penetrated mainly their legs and lower abdomen. Removing the fragments was a new problem for me and my orderlies, and one we needed to solve quickly to avoid the wounds becoming infected and developing into tropical ulcers.

One bloke in camp happened to be a surgical instrument maker by trade, and with him he was still carrying a small set of metal files and tools as well as a pictorial catalogue from Allen and Hanbury (a famous London-based surgical instrument firm). After examining his catalogue, I asked this fellow if he could fashion me a special pair of forceps with loops on the end, so I could probe into a wound, forcing it open to remove the fragment. He managed to pinch some scrap steel out on the Railway and made me an excellent instrument which I used daily. Among so many men in camp we had access to qualified experts in a wide range of fields, and all of us became skilled in the art of improvisation. Every problem was seen as a challenge to find a solution, and another opportunity to keep our minds active.

On 5 April, the Anglo-American (British and American) Force, under Captain Fitzsimmons, arrived from the 14 Kilo camp, along with a Dutch doctor, Captain Hekking, and an interpreter. These men had commenced line laying at the 14 Kilo camp, making progress at the rate of one and a half to two kilometres each day. Their sick created an extra load on the RAP staff, and also on our medical supplies, but we were glad to see the Yanks. A couple of their men were from the Bronx and on sick parade they always offered entertaining explanations for their ailments. My favourite was: 'Doc, da guts has gone on da bum again' — meaning dysentery.

With intense *speedo! speedo!* pressure for faster labour on the Railway, the Japanese demanded that two of my orderlies, Pinkey Rhodes and Don Booth, join the working parties. In camp, Jim Armstrong remained my sole orderly and the only other help I received was from those men marked 'No Duty' for a day. Jim worked harder than any man I have ever known. The sick were becoming sicker and, with no hospital accommodation available on site, patients were scattered throughout the camp, making it near impossible to attend adequately to them all. I ran four sick parades a day, one before breakfast for the 'new' sick, one in the morning for Anderson Force 'old' sick, one in the afternoon for Williams Force 'old' sick and then one in the evening when the men returned from work for those who had become ill or injured during the day. I was seeing over 350 men each day, including a case of smallpox among the British troops, along with other suspect cases. Naito refused to allow me to evacuate any of the sick to the hospital at Retpu (30 Kilo camp), so we were forced to isolate the smallpox cases some distance from the camp, in an old tent.

Working flat out proved to be a blessing. My job continued to provide me with a refuge from mental suffering: I escaped into my work. My days consisted of moving from one patient to the next, negotiating with guards in between, and then collapsing into our hut late at night for a few hours' sleep before doing it all again the next day. Seldom did I have free moments to contemplate our fate or become nostalgic with thoughts of home; if I did have a rare break, I tried to spend it either reading books from our still active mobile library, or discussing life and literature with my mate John Shaw, whose wise words always sustained and cheered me.

Physically though, life in captivity was starting to take its toll. I was suffering recurrent diarrhoea, sometimes passing more than twenty motions a day. Diarrhoea was a constant for all men all the time, but it varied in severity. A 'normal' case usually involved about ten motions per day, a severe dose about twenty or more. With all men suffering malnutrition none of us could afford to be losing the scant vitamins available in our pathetic rations. Diarrhoea could lead to dehydration and with no washing facilities and many men unable to make it to the latrines in time, it only added to our problems with hygiene and sanitation. Sometimes, if one of the men was looking to escape labour, he'd report to me on sick parade claiming to have a severe bout of diarrhoea in an attempt to be marked 'No Duty' for a day. I later discovered some were placing bets to see who could 'toss the

Doc', and I quickly developed a sixth sense for knowing who was lying and who was telling the truth. One fellow in particular, who shall remain nameless, reported to me on parade one morning, not looking too much the worse for wear. When I asked him how many motions he had passed, he answered: 'Twenty-seven, sir'. Immediately I was suspicious — in my experience, most men lost count after twenty.

'Twenty-seven motions?' I said. 'You'd better stay here in the RAP. And you're far too sick to be walking back and forth to the latrine, you can use this.' I handed him a tin hat to use as his 'pot'. His face went pale and I knew I had caught him out. When I returned to the RAP a few hours later, the tin hat was empty. My patient offered no explanation, just a shrug and a guilty face. I marked him as 'Duty' for the next day.

ABOUT TWO WEEKS AFTER being attacked by Nagatomo, Naito more or less recovered from his injuries and he was back to his inebriated worst, indulging in binge drinking sessions which lasted days at a time. Naito caused considerable anxiety not only to us but also his own guards, who despised him almost as much as we did. I remember one particular morning when one of Naito's guards approached him to deliver a message. Failing to salute his master correctly before relaying the message, the guard was sent back to the guardhouse, some 200 metres away, and ordered to return, at the double, and deliver the message in the approved fashion. The guard's repeat performance, however, still did not satisfy Naito and, after a further three attempts, the guard was so exhausted he collapsed at his master's feet. Naito stood up, and, using the scabbard of his sword, bashed the guard around the neck and shoulders while he was still on the ground, beating him mercilessly until he stopped moving.

Naito harassed his guards to such an extent that frequently many 'went bush', disappearing into the jungle for brief respite.

On occasions when he actually noticed his guards were missing, Naito formed his own search parties, usually consisting of half a dozen of the guards still in camp. In a drunken rage that bordered on dementia, he would take his party of guards on a training exercise, including rifle drills and charging with bayonets. One day Naito led his guards on an attack on a hill adjacent to our camp — on top of which were situated our latrines. Naito ordered his men to 'capture' the latrines, forcing his men to charge at them with bayonets while screaming three '*Banzais*' for the Emperor. Watching from camp, we were astounded by Naito's absurd military achievement on 'dunny hill'. One bloke standing near me exclaimed, 'Did you see that, Doc?' in pure disbelief. I could only nod. Behind Naito's back, we awarded him the 'Order of the Flying Kite' — he was clearly becoming progressively insane.

In between his binges, Naito displayed rare moments of what I could only construe to be alcoholic remorse, when his behaviour was almost human. The afternoon of 15 April is one I will never forget. A summary order arrived from Naito demanding the immediate presence of Colonel Anderson, Colonel Williams, Captain Fitzsimmons, Captain Hekking, Captain Drower (our interpreter) and me at his office. Knowing Naito was already 'on it', we anticipated trouble. Collecting our statistics and records of sickness and workers, we quickly agreed on excuses we could offer to explain the number of men we had marked 'No Duty' over the past few days.

Filled with dread, we arrived at Naito's office to find that his table had been dressed with colourful sarongs. Naito was sitting at the head of the table and, upon our entrance, he staggered to his feet to welcome us.

'I order you to enjoy yourselves. This is a party.'

We watched with nervous scepticism as Naito's subordinates set the table with a plate and spoon for each of us, and then proceeded to produce green peas from a tin, followed by tinned pears, cucumber, onions, peanut toffee, brandy and cigarettes. None of us said a word, suspicious of his motive.

'Sit!' he ordered. Also at the table was Sergeant Shimojo, a new arrival in camp. The camp commanders, Anderson and Williams, sat near Naito at the head of the table, while I took my place near Hekking, closer to Shimojo. (Relations between Anderson and me had remained strained since our confrontation, but in public, we never let our differences show; we maintained a normal commanding officer–RMO appearance at all times.) I glanced at Naito; his nose and cheeks glowed a ruddy red, the face of a drinker.

In the early stages, to prevent Naito from drinking more, we considered it our duty to consume the two bottles of brandy on display as quickly as possible. But as soon as the bottles were finished, Naito sent his servants off to fetch more. The supply seemed to be limitless and we realised this was going to be a 'session'. With our bodies unaccustomed to alcohol and such a variety of food, the brandy quickly affected me. I felt light-headed, giddy. Colonel Anderson and Colonel Williams drank very little, so it was left to us younger and more foolish men to hold the fort and try to keep pace with Naito and Shimojo, who insisted we keep drinking with them. Conversation at the table was unnaturally polite. We spoke only when spoken to; after all, living with Naito was like waiting for an explosion: we knew that ceremonial humiliation or violence could erupt at any moment.

By the time the party eventually terminated, at about 2000 hours, except for Anderson and Williams, we were all 'full'. Beneath the table was a large pool of brandy, poured directly from our glasses onto the mud floor when we just couldn't drink any more. We returned to our billets in silence; all of us were beyond questioning the rationality of Naito's behaviour. He had the personality of Jekyll and Hyde, and we were thankful to have escaped what we expected to be a bashing. We accepted the evening for what it was, nodded goodnight to one another and fell into an exhausted sleep on our bamboo platforms.

TOWARDS THE END OF our time at Kunknitkway, I noticed that Captain Bill Drower had a small ulcer on his ankle. He'd been walking with it for days so I bullied him into staying in bed for a day to force him to rest. Later that same morning, Naito sent for Drower on a trivial matter. Drower, by now in some pain, wrote a short note of apology to Naito and suggested that the Korean messenger might be able to do what was required. Drunk yet again, Naito was enraged by Drower's note. When he inspected the worksheets of the day and discovered that Drower had originally been marked down as 'Duty', he immediately sent for me and Colonel Anderson. Naito demanded to know why we were concealing sick men, accusing us of marking sick men as workers so they would still receive full rations. After a stormy but very short interview, we were dismissed. This was just the beginning of what would become a very strange, almost farcical day.

A little later, Naito emerged from his headquarters and demanded to see Drower. After inspecting Drower's ankle, Naito, determined to seek retribution, declared that the ulcer was smallpox and immediately ordered Drower to be transferred to the isolation tent outside our camp. Accompanied by an armed guard, Naito escorted Drower to his new accommodation, ordering that he be placed next to a smallpox patient who was in the most awful stage of the disease — covered in weeping sores. He had just been bathed and the basin containing his dirty water had been left near the entrance to the tent. Naito, now satisfied that Drower had been put to bed in just the right spot, pointed to the basin and demanded to be doused with what he assumed was 'disinfectant'. Dr Hekking, who was also present, tried to tell Naito that there was no disinfectant but Naito, in his intoxicated state, again pointed to the basin of cloudy water — which looked not unlike a creosote solution, sometimes used as a powerful antiseptic. Dr Hekking complied immediately, with rather more enthusiasm than was warranted. (Despite Hekking's efforts, Naito's vaccination proved too much for the invading organisms.)

When Naito returned to his office, I arranged for Drower's bedding, clothes, eating irons and other odds and ends to be taken to him. Then, as if on cue, at the precise moment the bedding was being carried over the only exposed patch of ground between Drower's old billet and his new one, Naito reappeared. Livid, he ordered the bedding and Drower's personal belongings be brought to a space outside his office, and then, once again, he sent for Colonel Anderson and me.

Brandishing his revolver, Naito told Colonel Anderson what a 'bad man' he was to falsify the work sheets, and then accused me of being a 'bad boy' for concealing such a nasty disease as smallpox.

'It is not smallpox,' I said in a quiet voice. 'An ulcer. Needs rest.'

Naito, uninterested in my response, sent us outside with one of his stooges, a Korean guard, who was ordered to beat us up. With Naito still inside, the guard, who hated his superior, decided to go easy on us. He kicked us about a little and then, to make Naito think he was doing his job satisfactorily, screamed at us. Anderson was allowed to leave and I was ordered, as RMO, to personally supervise the burning of Drower's bedding and all his effects.

With the assistance of a couple of our lads, I gathered straw and dead grass and piled it on top of the bedding while, at the same time, sneaking out from under the blankets such valuable items as Drower's diary and personal trinkets. Naito had two sentries posted by us all the whole time so we could only take what we could shove beneath our scant clothing. Just as we were about to set fire to the grass, Naito's batman appeared and, to show his hatred for Naito, he offered to remove Drower's clothing, blankets and other personal items for safekeeping — which he did.

Naito, whose timing was proving to be impeccable on this particular day, appeared just as the flames began to burn brightly. Unfortunately he was not too drunk to realise that a lot of articles were missing from the flaming pile. He demanded that I tell him where the items were. I raised my head, blinking quickly, and pointed out — quite lamely — that I had been engaged in collecting dead grass at the time and had no idea what had happened to them (it was the best I could come up with on the spot). Not surprisingly, my response did not hold water, so I further pointed out that Naito's own sentries had been present the whole time and suggested that he might ask them what had happened. Not wanting to lose face, Naito gracefully backed down and insisted that his batman and I should search the camp in an endeavour to find where the articles had betaken themselves. We both left at the double and after an 'extensive search', managed to find an old pair of shorts, a couple of torn singlets and a few other bits and pieces kindly donated by amused prisoners of war who had been watching events unfold. We returned these to the impatiently waiting Naito, who ordered us to throw them into the flames. He waited until the last of the flames had died out before ordering me to his headquarters for the third time that day.

I followed Naito inside. His rubber-soled boots scuffed against the floorboards; his face flushed with anger. Jerking his head, he again told me I was a very, very 'bad boy'. For more than half an hour he lectured me, threatening all sorts of punishment — including being beaten or put in isolation — his revolver twirling around and around on his forefinger the whole time. Every minute seemed to drag; I watched his lips form an alcoholic grin, broad and stupid. My hackles rose, but I remained silent, cautious not to further inflame his rage. There was nothing I could do but wait for whatever punishment would be forthcoming.

'Reform!' he growled, banging a fist on the table like an angry judge in possession of his court. He then ordered a Japanese guard to beat me again.

Leading me outside, the guard, a fairly quiet little chap, endeavoured to convey to me in broken English that this was going to hurt him more than it was going to hurt me. Like hell, I thought. I took off my specs and held them in one hand and waited for the guard to explode. But just as he was about to carry out his orders, one of the older Korean guards, reportedly a Christian, arrived on the scene. Pleased to be excused from his task, the Japanese guard disappeared. The Korean screamed loudly at me and proceeded to punch a fist into the palm of his own hand repeatedly — *thwack, thwack, thwack* — right next to my face, creating the impression that I was being thoroughly beaten: flesh on flesh. No matter how much the guards despised Naito, it was very rare for them to come to our aid, and now I had received two reprieves in one day — a miracle!

The Korean guard maintained his theatrical beating for some time, to avoid suspicion from Naito, who was still inside his hut, before shooing me away with his outstretched hands. I obeyed, fleeing the scene with far more speed than dignity; my heart racing as fast as my scrawny legs could carry me.

CHAPTER TEN

A NEW KILLER

Kunknitkway (26 Kilo camp) to Anarkwan (45 Kilo camp),
then to Taunzan (60 Kilo camp)
April–July 1943

We departed Kunknitkway on 23 April — Good Friday. Before leaving camp, we received a visit from a Japanese doctor, Higuchi, who allowed us to be vaccinated against cholera. I was surprised and grateful for the vaccine but questioned if it had been properly stored (refrigerated); if not, it could well prove to be useless. Higuchi permitted me to vaccinate most of my men, but not before he had carried out some himself, wiping his needle 'clean' with his fingers in between each injection![1] I boiled water in a billy can over a fire and sterilised the syringe and needles inside a perforated tobacco tin.

We spent the rest of the morning squatting on the hot red clay soil near the Railway line, awaiting orders from the Japanese. The sky was hazy with heat, the sun burning our bare skin. Days of waiting were always hard on the men; it gave them more time to let their minds wander to thoughts of home. I moved among the crowd, checking on the sick. While there was certainly no such thing recognised as counselling in those days, I also saw it as my duty as RMO to notice if a man seemed particularly down in the dumps. Often, just by stopping to say hello to a bloke I would soon discover it was his wife's birthday or their wedding anniversary, or some other auspicious occasion, and initiating a chat sometimes seemed to help him get things off his chest and pass the time.

In the afternoon a train finally arrived. Exhausted and thirsty from the heat, we clambered aboard the flat, open steel trucks (drawn by motor trucks converted to run on rails). I helped the sick onboard and then assisted other officers in checking who was aboard and who wasn't. We had just settled into our positions, waiting for the train to depart, when Naito staggered onto the scene, a guard on either side, propping him up; he was so inebriated he could not stand unsupported.

Armed with a sword hanging from his left hip and a revolver on his right, he ordered everybody to detrain immediately. As the representative of His Imperial Highness, Naito was insisting that he be the first to board our train. Hardly surprised by his antics, we scrambled from the trucks, helping the sick on their way. We then watched Naito board the train, still assisted by his two goons, and take his place in his specially reserved seat. It was no more than a plank resting across a couple of petrol drums; nonetheless, he considered it his rightful throne. A smug grin on his face, he ordered us to board the train all over again.

As the train pulled out, loaded with the first batch of POWs, including me, Naito suddenly rose from his plank to his unsteady feet and waved in a girlish fashion to those remaining on the platform. We were delighted to see our lads return the wave in true Australian style, including certain variations that could have been mistaken for the 'V for Victory' sign. Naito, thrilled by such a hearty response, expressed his satisfaction by throwing a few bits of pineapple to men near his 'throne', as if tossing fish to seals.

ANARKWAN CAMP, IN COMPARISON to Kunknitkway, was almost pleasant: it was situated by a wide river with magnificent hills in the background and green jungle scenery intervening. The huts were in decent condition despite being full of bugs and lice, and we were allocated a separate hut for an RAP and hospital that would accommodate some 50 patients. But while the state of our camp was an improvement, the physical condition of the men remained alarming. For the last three nights at Kunknitkway, Naito had forced men to work all night on the Railway — now they were almost dead on their feet. On arrival, we were given orders that 80 per cent of men had to go to work, allowing for 10 per cent camp workers and 10 per cent sick. I could not come up with enough fit men to meet the required quota. Naito sent all men marked 'Light Duties' out to the Railway regardless, where he forced them to labour for almost 24 hours straight.

On our third day in camp we were rejoined by Fitzsimmons Force, but they were without Dr Hekking, who remained at Kunknitkway to look after the smallpox cases, including our interpreter, Captain Bill Drower. (Remarkably, Drower still hadn't contracted the disease, but Naito, in his vengeful way, insisted on leaving him in the isolation tent even then.) With Hekking absent, I inherited Fitzsimmons Force sick parades in addition to those of Anderson and Williams Forces. I was now responsible for some 1600 men, seeing 450 to 500 sick per day.

Fitzsimmons Force was an undisciplined bunch, consistently failing to report in an orderly column, but gradually I trained them to realise that a sick parade was still a formal parade. Reporting in numerical order meant we could check each man against the roll book and with so many sick to attend to it was important to run the parades as efficiently as possible for the benefit of all. The 'new' sick of all forces were seen before breakfast, Anderson Force 'old' sick and hospital patients were seen during the morning, Williams Force 'old' sick were seen after lunch and the Anglo-American 'old' sick were seen after tea. When the workers returned, somewhere around 2200 or 2300 hours, I treated any injuries and the 'new' sick. There were already 60 patients cooped up in the camp hospital and the Japanese refused to allow any to be evacuated to Retpu Hospital.

I was appalled by the condition of the British troops. They still failed to grasp the concepts of hygiene and sanitation, and scabies was rife among their men. Antagonism between the British and Australian troops was ever-present. If any of our blokes caught one of the Brits intentionally defecating anywhere but in the latrines — a not uncommon occurrence — he would rub the offender's nose in his own faeces. I remember one night at a camp we shared with the Brits where we had actually built bamboo stalls around our slit-trench latrines, one of our men was going about his business when a Pom approached and sang out, 'Anyone in there?' Out of the dark our bloke grunted, 'yes'. The Pom then backed in to the stall and let go all over him. When the Australian abused him, the Pom said, 'Terribly sorry old chap, I thought you said "no".'

THE RANKS OF THE sick continued to mount each day as the Japanese pushed men to labour harder and longer on the Railway. Food rations remained hopeless: in the main, there were now only dollops of rice, minimal protein and almost no vitamins or fresh food. If we received stew with our rice it was always watery and barely flavoured the rice. Lucky was any man who found more than a piece of vegetable or shred of meat (often rotten) in his dixie. The men were now so thin their ribs protruded from their wasted bodies. It was frightening to watch their physical deterioration. I was convinced that many could not keep going for much longer, existing on a grossly deficient diet, endless labour, disease and, on top of all this, worsening physical violence, which escalated to an all-new level at the end of April.

It started out on the Railway when a Japanese ganger bashed AB (able-bodied seaman) Freddy Mills, of HMAS *Perth* in Williams Force. His offence? Driving a spike into a sleeper at an angle instead of straight down. The ganger had then gone running to a Japanese officer, falsely claiming that he had been hit by Mills. In response, the Japanese officer also bashed Mills. Lieutenant Lloyd Burgess, a Williams Force officer in charge of Mills' working party, calmed the situation temporarily by explaining it had all been a misunderstanding owing to a language problem, but for the rest of the afternoon Mills suffered further beatings from every guard who walked past him.

Later that day, when the men returned to camp, Mills, along with Lieutenant Burgess and another officer, was ordered into the jungle by Japanese guards. There he was struck with the butt of a rifle in an attempt to force him to confess to hitting the Japanese ganger, and his jaw was broken. While beatings happened daily, breaking a man's jaw was an all-new low; yet another line had been crossed. What's more, one of the guards then fired a bullet right above Mills' head, at which point Lieutenant Burgess and the other officer — who, up until then, had been able to do little to help — insisted that they be allowed to take Mills back to camp. Mills was brought directly to me, and I wasted no time in admitting him to our hospital. He was a bloody mess. Purple bruising covered his cheeks, also beneath his tongue and on the floor of his mouth. He was having difficulty breathing normally and he couldn't talk or swallow.[2]

These events took place in the absence of Naito, otherwise the end result for Mills could have been even worse. Colonel Anderson and Captain Fitzsimmons had already left for Thanbyuzayat, accompanied by Naito, to attend a camp commanders' conference. When they returned in early May — without Naito — they told us of the incredible events that had taken place at base camp.

High-ranking Japanese officers from the military's Propaganda Department had been taking moving pictures of the prisoners at play, at work and in hospital at Thanbyuzayat, determined to show the world just how well we POWs were being cared for (further proof that they knew how they *should* have been treating us.) Cartloads of vegetables, rice and fruit were brought into the camp for the occasion, and the hospital dispensary was stacked with drugs and dressings. Of course, as soon as the photographs were taken, all the supplies were removed. During a big 'do' on the football field, Naito, while making a speech of welcome to the visiting dignitaries, passed out on the platform. He was immediately transferred to Moulmein Hospital suffering from a 'cerebral haemorrhage'. We had finally seen the last of Naito.

AS THE HEALTH OF men further deteriorated in what was becoming an increasingly cheerless camp, morale started to become strained. With the privilege of rank, officers almost unquestionably had a better chance of survival than others, primarily because they did not have to labour on the Railway. The risk of embitterment from men towards officers, especially as *speedo! speedo!* pressure increased, could have been very real, but men such as Colonel Williams ensured this was not true for our group. Williams displayed his own unique brand of unbreakable courage — perhaps never more so than on 8 May.

That morning, a Japanese film crew had arrived in our camp to capture even more footage to be used for propaganda purposes. All prisoners of war were ordered to dress in shorts and a shirt for the filming, but of course most of the men had none. The Japanese quartermaster, knowing that the film crew wanted to record the sounding of reveille, ordered Williams to provide the film crew with a bugler. Colonel Williams advised that he would do so; however, with the bugler out working on the Railway, the film crew would have to wait until he returned to camp that night.

Recognising that the quartermaster did not seem to understand, Colonel Williams also repeated his response to the cameraman, who indicated he didn't mind. Just before midnight, the film crew again, via the quartermaster, demanded the presence of the bugler, and Colonel Williams had to explain once more that the man in question was still out at work on the Railway.

Sergeant Shimojo, newly appointed as our camp commander and keen to impress his visiting film crew, severely reprimanded both Colonels Anderson and Williams, demanding that they should each know the whereabouts of every one of their men at all times (all 1467 of them!).[3] Williams, never one to shy away from confrontation, told Shimojo that he had already advised both the quartermaster and the cameraman of the whereabouts of the bugler.

Incensed, Shimojo accused Williams of lying and, as punishment, ordered him to stand outside the guardhouse bareheaded, in later what would be the blazing sun and, later again, the pouring rain. Throughout the day, Williams was advised by guards that the punishment would end if he would apologise to Shimojo. True to form, Williams not only refused to apologise but told the guards the entire matter was the fault of the quartermaster, cameraman and Shimojo. Whenever a guard walked past he took a swing at the colonel or gave him a swift kick with his boot. Given nothing to eat or drink but a single mug of broth, Williams stood at attention for the term of his punishment, which came to an end after 26 hours of agony: it was a magnificent effort by a brave man.[4]

Courage of the like displayed by Williams provided a huge boost to the spirits of the men. By continually taking a stance against the Japanese, always at great personal cost, Williams was an inspiration. The fact that he never gave up or gave in, filled the men with confidence that his presence made a very real difference to their odds of surviving. Williams' leadership consistently reminded all of us that dignity and justice were always worth fighting for, at any cost.

THE FOLLOWING DAY, WITHOUT warning, we were suddenly ordered to move to Taunzan (60 Kilo camp). We could smell this camp long before we arrived. Indescribably filthy, we immediately christened it 'Faecole'. We were not only greeted with piles of rubbish and faeces but also with the corpses of scores of emaciated Burmese. Many were bloated and thick with flies, laid out like fish at a market not far from our huts. The foul stench of decomposing bodies made us retch. Further back on the Railway, we had, at times, felt anger towards the local Burmese for their lack of hygiene, frustrated that they were carrying germs into our camps. But that had quickly passed. We now felt genuine empathy for them. Our lives were miserable but theirs were obviously worse: they had been captured and tortured in their own land and were dying daily.

Shimojo sent men to work on the Railway immediately, while those remaining in camp — the sick, supervised by some officers — were left to clean the camp and remove the corpses. Immediate burial of the bodies was essential to prevent the spread of disease, the urgency even greater in a tropical climate, where decay sets in so quickly and flies are active in their millions. Our men carried the dead to a crude cemetery where the Burmese had already buried between 150 and 200 bodies in shallow graves. The bodies were buried with respect but without ceremony.

As the days passed, more and more Burmese lost their lives. The possible cause of their deaths created considerable anxiety among us all. Were they dying from malnutrition and exhaustion, or was it a more serious killer: smallpox, plague, malaria or cholera? My worst fears were confirmed about two weeks after our arrival at Taunzan.

One of the Japanese engineers was first to die, followed by one of our own men, Gunner F.G. Dare (of the 2/10th Field Regiment). Prior to his death, Dare had not been feeling well for three or four days, but had worked regardless — during this time, the Japanese had insisted that almost 100 of our sick men be sent to work on the Railway and perform the same work for the same duration of time as the 'fit' workers. The night before he died, I saw him at about 1900 hours, when I administered 1 cc of pestis (plague) vaccine and noted that he appeared to be in fairly 'normal' health, by current standards. At 2400 hours he complained of slight abdominal pain before passing four small watery motions and vomiting a little. Initially, I suspected an attack of malaria. When I saw him again at about 0400 hours, his pain warranted an injection of one-quarter of a grain of morphia from my personal kit and a stomach sedative. By 0900 hours he displayed the picture of severe prostration, dehydration, cramps in the legs and abdomen, and devitalised skin, yellow–grey in colour. Heat and massage were applied to relieve the cramps but without much success. His face muscles went into minor spasm, producing a mild 'risus sardonicus' (a sardonic smile, almost diagnostic of cholera), a very disturbing sight. Just after 1300 hours, he suddenly collapsed and was dead in a matter of twenty minutes. It had to be cholera.

A Japanese laboratory technician, in camp taking rectal smears from Japanese guards who feared for their own safety, inspected two more of our men, both of whom I also suspected might have the disease. Positive cultures confirmed my clinical diagnosis.

There were two types of cholera: 'wet', the most common form, and 'dry' (also known as *cholera sicca*). The wet variety made dysentery look like constipation, with men passing what we called 'rice-water stools' up to once every fifteen minutes. In the dry form, there was very little diarrhoea but the results were even more dramatic: a man could die within hours after only a few bowel actions. In very simple terms, in both cases the cholera germs inside the body developed toxins which spread rapidly, causing dehydration. Death from severe dehydration could result in a frighteningly short period of time, just a few hours. Highly infectious, cholera was mainly spread through contaminated water and food. It could be controlled or prevented by adequate booster injections of properly stored vaccine, to ensure that immunity did not wear off. I still held grave fears about the quality of the vaccine we had been administered back at Kunknitkway.

With suspected cholera cases formally verified, our guards, in a state of panic, were suddenly prepared to oblige most of our requests. In addition to our existing hospital, we took control of a disused stable which we converted into an isolation 'hospital', complete with fireplaces, latrines, mosquito nets and a series of separate raised decks, each carrying four to six patients at intervals of about three metres. These were so arranged that the patients with suspected cholera, dysentery and severe diarrhoea could be formed into small separate groups, making for ease within isolation when any was found to be bacteriologically or clinically positive with cholera. We staffed this hospital with some orderlies from Anderson Force and some from Williams Force, with Jim Armstrong and Pinkey Rhodes in charge.[5] All were outstanding in their dedication, putting their own lives at risk to care for sick comrades: it was an astounding example of a very special type of courage.

The Japanese, upon request, gave us quicklime and some form of phenol to use as antiseptics. Sanitation in the isolation hospital was maintained at as high a standard as possible in primitive conditions. The isolation hospital was out of bounds to all except those volunteer orderlies who lived in a separate area within the hospital, and Jim Armstrong, Pinkey Rhodes and me. I did, however, turn a blind eye when I saw movement in the long grass between camp and the hospital: it usually meant that either Colonel Williams was creeping in to visit his men or Padre 'Pessimistic Pete' Smith — 'Don't worry, the war will be all over in five or ten years, certainly fifteen' — was on his way to shave the very sick and offer spiritual comfort. These two men took full hygiene precautions, scrubbing their hands and dipping them in chlorine solution before and after visits. The psychological value of their visits to the sick far outweighed the added risk of infection. The presence of Williams and Pete helped the men to maintain hope, to keep fighting; they reminded them that those in camp had not given up on them.

Watching Padre Pete with the sick, I sometimes envied the believers for their profound faith, simply for the great comfort it so obviously offered. My own views on religion had remained unchanged, but at times during captivity I coveted their certainty, their understanding of their own place in the world. I often thought of my mother's words: 'Trust in God and fear no man' — but as far as I was concerned, there was no sign of God in the jungles of Burma.

Treatment of cholera was severely limited, although I was grateful I still had bottles of Ringer's solution (a saline mixture with minerals added, used to aid hydration) — the only useful item I had been left with when my pannier had been looted way back at Tavoy. Jim, Pinkey and I spent long nights at the isolation hut, endeavouring to administer the Ringer's solution intravenously to patients, often while contending with plagues of flying ants. Our improvised IV apparatus consisted of a bottle with the bottom knocked off, a 10 cc syringe barrel as a drip control, stethoscope tubing to carry the solution and a piece of sharpened brass tubing as a cannula.

On one occasion, Jim and I only managed to administer 30 cc to a patient when we had to stop, owing to a far from satisfactory hypodermic (fine bore) needle. We prepared a wider bore needle, made from a piece of copper tubing 'salvaged' from one of the Japanese trucks, which we hoped would do the trick for the remaining dosage. During the infusion process, overcome by the heat, I keeled over. I was grateful that Colonel Williams had chosen that precise moment to visit his men. He kindly assisted

Jim in keeping the infusion going until I regained my feet. Our workload was becoming increasingly impossible: aside from cholera, we also experienced a malaria epidemic. There were 80 'textbook' cases in eight days, featuring the typical rigors, fever, sweating, pains in the eyes, knees and other joints. Fortunately, we had an adequate, though finite, supply of quinine for treatment, again courtesy of the panic-stricken guards, but in terms of medical staff, there were never enough hours in the day.

Throughout the rest of the camp, our well-established hygiene discipline was further tightened. In addition to never drinking unboiled water and sterilising dixies, I asked men to focus on the four 'Fs' — food, flies, fingers and faeces — along with water, the most common channels for transmitting cholera. The wet season only heightened the risk of men contracting the disease. The weather was mostly hot with days of rain; it was very wet underfoot, our handmade clogs sinking in the mud. I banned men from bathing in the now swollen river that cut its way through beautiful jungle undergrowth near the camp. They were to bathe in camp, using boiled water when possible — being careful never to get their heads wet.

Extreme caution was also taken in transporting food from the main camp to the isolation hospital. The isolation orderlies placed sterilised, empty buckets on the boundary to the main camp and then walked back towards the isolation hospital, ensuring they were at least a few metres from the boundary. The main camp kitchen orderlies then approached and poured food, usually rice and watery stew, into the isolation buckets and then left. Once the kitchen orderlies had departed, the isolation orderlies then collected the buckets and distributed the food. These isolation orderlies took the greatest of care to ensure they never came into contact with those in the main camp.

In retrospect, Jim and I realised that most in the camp had probably experienced a mild abortive attack of cholera a couple of days before we had diagnosed it as such. Many, including me, had passed a few 'extra brisk', watery motions which had ceased in a few hours — probably thanks to the cholera injections we had received at Kunknitkway. I shuddered when I thought of what might have been. We hoped that those of us who had not by then succumbed to cholera had the necessary immunity to protect us from the disease that could strike terror into the hearts of even the bravest of men.

AT THE END OF May, Bill Drower and surgeon Syd Krantz arrived in camp, bringing with them 100 yen, courtesy of the International Red Cross, and 96 eggs purchased from our own Red Cross fund (which was still being financed by a portion of the pay we received from the Japanese). We were very pleased to see Bill Drower alive and well — we hadn't seen him since Naito abandoned him in the smallpox tent at Kunknitkway.[6] With close to 100 very sick men in our two hospitals, the supply of eggs and cash was a godsend. The money enabled us to make an excellent canteen purchase, all of which was allocated to the sick, including, among other items, 400 eggs, two pineapples, and five chickens.

The day after the purchase, the menu for the sick included eggs, custard, orange juice, chicken broth, and oxtail soup. Our cooks were masters of economy, spinning out the pineapple supply for as long as possible by scraping the pulp from the skins, and then boiling it with *chindegar* to make syrup. This food, rich in protein and vitamins, was desperately needed, and really did mean the difference between life and death for many of the sick.

On 8 June I celebrated my 27th birthday, sharing my last drop of brandy with John Shaw and Jim Armstrong. Our cooks produced a special 'cake' in my honour, complete with 'Happy Birthday, 27' iced on the top. It was an incredibly thoughtful gesture on the part of the cooks and, I suspected, the RAP staff. The cake, so called, was made from ground rice and *chindegar*, while the icing was made from *chindegar* and a finer grade of ground rice. It was a brief respite from more pressing concerns. Williams Force had departed the day before, bound for the 40 Kilo camp, leaving me a legacy of 50 of its sickest patients. One man looked like dying at any time and many others were desperately ill. Considering how many men needed to be attended to, including further cases of cholera, it didn't help that I was feeling wretched with yet another attack of severe diarrhoea. Not the birthday present I might have hoped for.

A week later Major Kerr returned from a trip to Thanbyuzayat, bringing news of the previous day's bombing by Allied forces. Six Liberators, the biggest flying craft he had ever seen, bombed the rail and road crossing just a few hundred metres from the camp boundary. Twelve POWs were killed and two wounded; while among the Burmese there were 50 killed and 100 wounded. While we were saddened by the loss of our men, we were also encouraged that perhaps British General Archie Wavell was active after all. Allied bombings continued at Thanbyuzayat throughout the rest of the month, causing a temporary stop to work on the Railway. Instead, work parties were engaged in repairing the rain-damaged roads. We were, by now, in the midst of the wet season and the rivers were in full spate, making it nearly impossible to get food supplies through to us from base camp. Fortunately, our camp was situated about two kilometres from a large food dump (depot) and, as a result, we received an extra issue of perishable foodstuffs which could not be carried to those further along the line. For two weeks we had plenty of rice and over 200 grams of meat per man per day, with a generous supply of onions, beans and lentils. We had a good scrounger as quartermaster: any beast left unattended in the vicinity of our camp or anywhere within view of our men along the road, soon found itself hanging in our kitchen. The Japanese were only too willing to cooperate, as long as they received the choicest cuts, but it suited us: there was always a limit to what 20 or 30 guards were capable of eating.

Malaria was still an enormous worry and looked likely to become an even greater one. Despite improved rations and some medical supplies, including a cholera booster vaccine, men continued to die. By the end of June, we had lost eight more of our men since Gunner Dare had succumbed to suspected cholera: four of these deaths were from cholera (bacteriologically confirmed), three from suspected or clinically confirmed cases of malaria, and the other from chronic amoebic dysentery.[7] Some died in the arms of the orderlies, who ensured their comrades' last moments were filled with compassion and tenderness. I cannot praise these men highly enough — they were truly the unsung heroes.

Morale dropped further during this time as men discovered that one of their mates, sometimes the man who slept alongside them at night, had died or returned a positive rectal smear. Strangely, though, as we watched friends dying around us, most of us believed 'it can't happen to me'— perhaps another form of denial that sustained much-needed inner strength.

By this stage, we had become accustomed to living in a closed world, one from which we couldn't break out and which Allied rescuers couldn't, it seemed, break into. Our world was one where there was no logic for why one man lost his life and another did not. Was I scared of contracting cholera? No. If it happened, it happened. While we were fully aware of the grim risks we faced, most of us had become quite fatalistic. The difficulty with such a mindset, though, was to recognise the difference between inevitability and the possibility of changing our situation. We all hoped we had the strength to endure whatever was inevitable — for example we could not alter the fact that we would remain in captivity until the end of the war — while also maintaining the courage to change anything about our circumstances which could be changed — after all, we still had control over our thoughts, we could still keep our minds busy. If we possessed the wisdom to recognise the difference between what we could and could not control, then we had a chance of finding a way to survive.[8]

My own response to the deaths of my men began to border on disengagement — it had to. Over the past year, I had learned to adapt. My emotions, little by little, became blunted, making me desensitised to some extent, so I could learn to view awful and uncontrollable events as everyday occurrences. We lived with the ugly anticipation that there were always likely to be worse days to come, and I was now a hard man to shock. Death had become no more than a part of our life, one which I did not ignore, but could not dwell upon.

In order to cope, I believe, most men surrounded themselves in their own personal and protective armour. Mine, as I have already written, was work, an almost obsessive sense of duty; for others it was humour or religious faith; and for nearly all us, it was the setting of a deadline: 'home by Christmas' or 'home for my wife's birthday', or some other date of personal significance. In establishing a mental goal to work towards we were focusing on a future life which we could anticipate living and, in the process, attempt to reject the reality of what we were experiencing, deferring our disappointment. Keeping an 'end point' in mind, even though deep down we knew it was artificial, gave us hope — one of the most powerful weapons in the limited armoury of defence we could own. If we were to not only survive but also remain sane, it was all we could do.

WILLIAMS FORCE RETURNED TO our camp in early July and we had to squeeze up to make room for them. Two days later we received 15,000 tablets of quinine, of which we were in desperate need. This supply, however, would provide half-courses for only 600 attacks, while we predicted somewhere between 1700 to

1800 attacks on the then current incidence. By now, I had also succumbed to suspected malaria, suffering fever, backache, headache and sweating, and I was off duty, as much as possible, from the end of June until early July.

Even if the majority of our men escaped cholera, how, I questioned, could they survive the 'killer cycle' of malaria, dysentery and beriberi on top of starvation, hard labour and acts of brutality, all the while watching comrades die around them? The position of all men was truly grim, made even worse on 7 July by a heartless 'blitz' on the sick by our keepers, who demanded 300 out of the combined forces of 1000 men be sent to work. It was difficult to find even 200 well enough to survive labour in their current state.

We lost two more men of Anderson Force over the next couple of days, one from a combination of malaria, dysentery and malnutrition; the other from cholera, dysentery and pellagra. At least another twenty men were in a similar or worse condition, but they were hanging on. All the convalescent cholera cases, except for one, had developed diarrhoea, and the daily increase in beriberi oedema — the feet of men ballooning — added further to our worries. Jaundice was almost universal in those suffering recurrent attacks of malaria, including me: I couldn't stand the smell of food for days while I was recovering.

We were due to leave camp on 13 July and I wondered how many of our men would survive another journey. Before the move, Colonel Anderson and I were again at odds over the state of the men's health. Our antagonism towards one another had not improved: ever since arriving at Taunzan, I had been lobbying him continuously, through a written report and several face-to-face encounters, in regard to hygiene within the camp and care of the sick. I just could not make sense of what I perceived to be a lack of action on his behalf, or his persistent belief that he could 'educate' the Japanese to change their ways. Back in June, I had formally requested further measures be taken to prevent malaria, including a concerted effort to remove all stagnant water, and Anderson had responded to my request, bizarrely, with: 'Mosquitoes must live, malaria is not serious.'[9] He insisted that we mustn't kill any living thing.

With our last confrontation still fresh in my mind, and undoubtedly his, I entered his headquarters to discuss, privately and officially, the matter of men marching to our next camp. I maintained that the majority were unwell, and not fit for the journey. He insisted that the 'men [were] now capable of marching if their temperatures were 103° to 104°F'[10] (just as they were in Africa in the First World War).

It was one thing for him to question my medical judgment, but quite another to push our men, who were clearly dangerously ill, beyond their human limits. For a moment I lost all control, blurting out: 'You can murder the men if you choose!'[11]

I could barely believe such words had come out of my own mouth. I waited for his fury, but Anderson, ever the gentleman, only responded to my outburst with silence; his face blank. By this stage, I believed our CO to be cracking mentally due to being under extreme personal stress and carrying the responsibility of so many men — it is the only explanation I can offer for his attitude towards the sick. I still respected him as a great man and as my commanding officer, but I failed to understand him.

On my part, I was exasperated and also feeling great stress, particularly with some of the men around me starting to suffer from dementia. One man was experiencing malarial semi-delirium, as well as a persecution complex that he was about to be shot for trading with the Burmese. His condition appeared to be early pellagral dementia — the third D of the dermatitis, diarrhoea, dementia, death sequence. Another of our men was heading the same way, beginning to experience delusions of time, place and position. Looking back, perhaps I, too, was starting to crack. I was truly terrified of what a pellagra epidemic that progressed to the dementia stage would mean for all of us: the prospect of a camp full of dementia patients was simply beyond contemplation.

Defeated, I saluted Anderson and left.

CHAPTER ELEVEN

DEATH CAMPS
Taunzan (60 Kilo camp) to Mizale (70 Kilo camp), to Apparon (80 Kilo camp)
July–August 1943

When rails had been laid up to the 68 Kilo peg, the guards ordered our men to pack up all heavy camp equipment. It was to be moved by rail from the 60 Kilo camp to the 68 Kilo mark, where the rail line finished; then the men would unload and carry everything the remaining two kilometres to Mizale (70 Kilo camp). It would have made more sense to allow the men to lay the rail all the way to the next camp, only a day or two more of work, but the bloody-minded guards preferred to watch starving men, swaying with fatigue, carry everything — *speedo! speedo!* — on foot. Considering all the work the Japanese needed done on the Railway, it seemed absurd to us that they couldn't see the logic in preserving our strength wherever possible, let alone giving us enough food and medicines, in order to create a larger, stronger and more productive labour force to satisfy their own requirements. But in their minds, we were just prisoners, 100 per cent expendable. If we died, so be it; they were confident they had access to a never-ending supply of slave labour.

While the so-called fit men travelled to Mizale, I stayed behind, along with the stretcher-bearers, to accompany the sick on their journey to the 55 Kilo camp hospital. (The Japanese had, without explanation, deemed that I was now allowed to evacuate the sick.) There were 41 stretcher-bearers and 114 sick. The guard in charge of this party, 'Boofhead' — an aggressive Korean *speedo* merchant and a hulk of a man — lunged at the stretcher-bearers with bamboo sticks and stabbed at their legs with his fixed bayonet while they loaded and unloaded patients. The cholera patients were the last to be moved, taken to the entraining point late in the afternoon when it was growing cold and drizzling with rain. One of the men from Williams Force died while waiting and had to be carried back to camp to be buried.

The 55 Kilo camp hospital was a soul-destroying sight: with no fit men in camp apart from medical orderlies, there was no one to attend to important duties such as cooking and hygiene. It's hard to convey just how grim a prisoner of war hospital can be. All around me the sick looked small, wasted; their muscles stringy and their skin pulled tight over prominent bones. The Japanese did not need to apply any other techniques of torture: through gross neglect alone they were already sentencing so many of these men to slow and painful deaths.

Conditions were so bleak I could not help feeling that I was signing the death warrant of my own lads when I evacuated them from our camp, but I had no option. It was almost impossible for us to carry our own sick on our numerous moves and there was always a chance that conditions may improve in a hospital camp (being so much closer to headquarters and supplies), whereas there was every indication that our conditions would only become worse along the Railway.

I returned to the 60 Kilo camp late that night, along with the stretcher-bearers and under the constant guard of Boofhead. We would be up early in the morning to rejoin the rest of our men at Mizale. I went to sleep on bamboo slats, my thoughts still with the sick men I had had to leave behind.

MIZALE (70 KILO CAMP) was the foulest camp we had experienced to date. The camp area was covered with slippery mud and slush from continual rain. Along with plagues of flies, biting sandflies hovered around us in their millions, their onslaught taking place at dusk. All night men slapped at their bare skin in an attempt to squash the bugs. In my diary I gave this camp a four-star 'filth rating'. It was extremely overcrowded, with 730 men forced into a wide and 100-metre-long hut. The men were packed in like matches in a matchbox: about sixteen men to each bay of four metres by three metres. By this time almost every man had obtained two empty rice or vegetable bags, which, with two bamboo poles threaded through each side and a spreader at each end, made serviceable Australian bushman-style camp beds. These beds were tied to four uprights and in many cases stacked three or four high.

The morning after our arrival, Boofhead organised a clean-up campaign involving every man in camp. A thorough job was done in a very short period of time due, in the main, to the guard's big bamboo sticks, which he used to issue a whirlwind of swipes to the heads and shoulders of men who weren't working quickly enough. Our main task was to remove all rubbish and clean and deepen drains in an attempt to remove the mud. Such a clean-up job would have taken several days under our own command, but we never would have resorted to Boofhead's depraved methodology.

For the RAP and hospital I was allocated only two bays, which was already inadequate; despite the fact that all the 'sick' had been sent to the 55 Kilo camp, many of the working men were also in very poor condition. One died of exhaustion soon after our arrival. It was a sudden blow to all of us as he had been in fairly good shape immediately prior to our departure, but the march had proved too much.

On my fourth day in camp, I discovered our two economic officers, Major Jim Jacobs (Anderson Force) and Major Ray Meagher (Williams Force), were due to visit the 55 Kilo, 45 Kilo and 40 Kilo camps. These two officers were personally responsible for paying the men, so were required to visit all detached units on a regular basis. Anxious to check on my sick men back at the 55 Kilo hospital, I managed to persuade the Japanese to allow me to accompany Jacobs and Meagher on their journey as a 'medical observer'. In turn, we were to be accompanied by 'The Storm Trooper', one of the most vicious and hated of all guards. Instead of regular bamboo, he favoured a much heavier metre-long wooden stick as his weapon of choice.[1]

We departed that same morning, the sick in camp being left in the capable and caring hands of Jim, Pinkey, Don and their team, with surgeon Syd Krantz to call on. We walked for the first kilometre before being picked up by a truck and driven for the next four kilometres. From there we had to travel a further five kilometres to the 60 Kilo site. The Storm Trooper, in his vast wisdom, insisted that we wait for five hours for a train to arrive to take us the remaining five kilometres to the 55 Kilo siding. It would have been much quicker to walk, but our opinion on the matter was obviously not requested. Being in charge of two majors and a captain, The Storm Trooper made it clear he was our 'big boss', shouting orders at us in front of other Japanese guards and the native Burmese to demonstrate his authority. Inexplicably, he was largely inoffensive towards us during the rest of the journey and did not resort to violence.

Conditions at the 55 Kilo camp hospital had not improved over the past week, there being some 1200 patients with a very tired and overworked Dr John Higgin to care for them. The poor beggar was worn to a frazzle and looked quite bewildered. The patients were divided into four large huts, with a further four huts containing a similar number of Dutch. The sight of that camp and the stench of the ulcer and dysentery wards were overwhelming. I was pretty hardened by then, but the rank smell of the ulcers very nearly made me vomit. The most seriously ill were isolated in a small hut known as 'the death house', from which six to eight men were being buried daily.

Inside the hospital, we saw Colonel Albert 'Bertie' Coates, a surgeon who was recovering from severe tropical typhus (for one month his temperature had ranged between 103 and 105 degrees Fahrenheit, his pulse rate exceeding 120). A veteran of the First World War, Coates had volunteered for duty in the Second World War at the age of 46. Following the disastrous Malayan campaign, he had cared for the sick and wounded in Sumatra before becoming a prisoner of war and being sent to the Burma–Siam Railway. Coates was renowned for his outstanding surgical work, and his influence permeated the hospital. He was well known for exhorting all men to eat their rice, every grain, no matter how sick they felt. 'Your passport home is in the bottom of your dixie,' he told them.

At the time, following the cholera epidemic, I was uncharacteristically depressed. When Coates and I were chatting, I had the nerve to complain to him that the experience I was getting of cholera, malaria, dysentery, beriberi and other tropical diseases was a waste of time, and that surely I would never see a single case of any of these when we returned home (I still expected to get home!). I will never forget his response.

'Rowley,' he said, 'you have learned something that few doctors ever learn, and it takes a lifetime of medicine for those who do. You have learned to know when a man is sick.'

I remember being unimpressed by his simple response, my face blank. It was not until some years later, when I had the opportunity to observe other doctors who had not been prisoners of war, that I understood and appreciated exactly what he had meant. I realised that I had developed a sixth sense, an instinctive gut feeling based on my experiences during captivity. I was able to recognise when a person was sick, even when they exhibited few symptoms and especially when a patient denied they required attention. Coates was a brilliant surgeon and a modest man. Having survived two world wars, he had an innate ability to see medical situations in a way that many others, me included, would take years to appreciate.

I was relieved to see my men from Anderson Force, as well as some from the 2/15th Field Regiment who had come down from the 105 Kilo camp. I could do little to help other than offer companionship and encouraging words. How, I wondered, could hope and optimism continue to exist alongside disease and death? I didn't know the answer. The injustice of watching young men suffering and losing their lives made me feel powerless but, more than anything, I was angry. Although I had to suppress any outward displays of outrage, locked inside my mind it still served as a fierce motivator: instead of feeling defeated, the fury I felt towards our keepers made me even more resolute not to give up or give in. In effect, anger played an important role as a self-defence mechanism, and there was never any shortage of incidents to trigger my internal rage: the starvation, disease and death of my men alone were enough to sustain enduring wrath and stubborn determination.

When I was ordered by The Storm Trooper to leave my men that afternoon, I privately resolved that the Japanese would never break me. I recognised then that freedom, in one sense, was a state of mind — and I was still free to *think* for myself, to retain control over my inner liberty. I only had two options: degenerate or survive. And once I acknowledged that the choice was mine, not that of my keepers, it was easy to make.

NOT LONG AFTER MY return to Mizale, there were several 'blitz' sick parades. The engineers demanded only 200 workers out of a combined force of nearly 900 men but still we could only produce 50, of whom only 30 were fit to work (according to the existing standards). Torrential rain had fallen during the previous weeks resulting in many washed-away roads, railways and bridges and the now scant working parties were forced to work all day and all night on repairs.

When the rails had been laid some 1200 metres short of the next camp, we were once more ordered to pack up all our equipment and travel by train from the 70 Kilo camp to the end of the rail line. It was 30 July. When the train stopped at the end of the line, yet again we were forced to lug all our heavy gear, as well as 70 stretcher cases, to our next camp, Apparon (80 Kilo camp).

Apparon was even worse than all its predecessors. Our huts, having previously been used as cattle yards by the Burmese, were covered in mud, slush and cow manure; the stench was nauseating. For the first few days we had difficulty in ejecting some of the remaining four-legged tenants — which, given the chance, we would have preferred to knock off and eat. Thankfully, the RAP and hospital were situated on a small hill some 400 metres distant — the one dry and almost clean spot in the camp area. There was a little stream running through the valley between the main camp and hospital area, and from it we drew our water. This necessitated a climb of about 200 metres up an extremely steep and slippery bank; the water being carried in four-gallon tins strung on poles.

Following an intense clean-up campaign in the main camp, again with the aid of big Korean-wielded sticks, we managed to establish some form of order but the inevitable mud and slush was beyond our control. All sorts of drains, stormwater channels and banks were built by our men in an endeavour to prevent the huts and our belongings from being washed away, but we still lived like neglected livestock — the floors of our huts covered in fifteen to twenty centimetres of mud. The heavy rain had washed away the bridge at the 60 Kilo peg, which resulted in our supplies of meat and rice not coming through. This was a constant problem during the wet season, and often, when we did finally receive the meagre meat rations, they would be full of maggots. During our early days of captivity, the cooks used to wash the maggots out, but now, with food so scarce, we decided that the maggots contained protein and the cooks just boiled them in with the meat.[2]

Down in the valley, about 800 metres from the main camp, was another hut, a so-called 'hospital'. It was, in effect, the dumping and burial ground for the sick of the No. 5 Branch in Thailand. The No. 5 Branch consisted of about 1000 Dutch, 450 Americans and 385 Australians. They had arrived from Java, via Singapore, and were located further up the line, near the Thailand border. The policy of the keepers of the No. 5 Branch was to retain — temporarily — the fit, and discard — permanently — the sick. When a man became ill, the keepers of the No. 5 Branch considered him to be a complete write-off: he was barely fed and given no medical attention. In this pathetic hospital, the diet of patients consisted of about 300 to 500 grams of rice per man per day, without salt, and flavoured only by grasses and greenery picked by the Dutch from the jungle. There was not one fit man in the camp who could act as a cook, or a medical orderly, or anyone to carry out any general camp duties. Sick men struggled to carry dead comrades to a graveyard nearby.

Major Syd Krantz and I secretly paid them a visit a couple of days after arriving at Apparon. There we met an American naval surgeon who was superintending a situation well beyond his control. We offered to inspect his patients, all of whom could only be classified as sick, dying or dead, and discovered that more than 200 had already been buried. Men lay back on their beds, their puny bodies lifeless, faces twisted with pain, eyes shut or staring fixedly at the *attap* roof. These were shattered men.

One of the men we examined, an Australian, had an extensive ulcer that stretched from his knee to his ankle. The sight of a tropical ulcer can be shocking, as if some kind of animal or acid has been eating its way through flesh, exposing the bone. On the surface, the dead tissue is black and dry, while the dying tissue is a yellowy brown, with pus and moisture visible even deeper into the wound. For the patient, the ulcerated area is exquisitely tender, causing intense burning pain, aching, itching and stinging. In this case, the patient's tibia had already died and a large sequestrum (a dead bone separated from living bone) was extruding. The stench was foul, like rotting meat. His leg desperately needed to be amputated if he had any hope of making it: without surgery, gangrene would rapidly produce fatal toxaemia.

Under the cover of darkness, we managed to sneak this man back to our own camp, accompanied by the American surgeon, whom we asked to assist us in the operation. Our patient, in agony, assured us he was willing to take the risk of amputation; he knew death was a certainty if he stayed in that hospital.

Our operating table was a bamboo platform inside the RAP, which although isolated was still close enough to the kitchen to enable a ready supply of boiling water for sterilisation. The American surgeon administered chloroform anaesthetic — courtesy of Syd's supplies — but of which we had very little, making the time factor in completing the amputation critical. Just as we were about to commence the operation, a couple of guards suddenly appeared, charging up to the RAP to see what was going on, ranting loudly, their eyes bulging. We froze: we knew the penalty for daring to perform such a procedure without their permission could be harsh. Yet when they came closer and saw the ulcer, the look of anger on their faces quickly turned to ghoulish interest. They stopped yelling and a tense silence filled the room. They indicated with hand gestures that we could continue, but only if they could watch; their sadistic tendencies obviously outweighing our crime.

Syd, experienced in amputations, explained how we would proceed. Because the patient's bone was already dead, the operation involved a disarticulation at the knee — in simple terms, we didn't need to cut through bone, only the ligaments and tendons that were still holding his joint together. Using Syd's instruments — a scalpel and artery forceps and not much else — together we amputated the leg in a matter of minutes, although it felt like much longer to us.

Throughout the operation, the guards didn't say a word, nor did they flinch; they were fascinated. Syd and I bandaged the patient's stump with strips of blankets sterilised in boiling water and within minutes the lad began to regain consciousness. He was groggy, mumbling words we couldn't understand and in extreme pain. I gave him morphia from my personal kit.

Almost a week after the amputation, the condition of our patient started to deteriorate considerably, due not to the effects of the operation but rather to a combination of neuritis, paralysis of the other leg, malaria, general toxaemia and exhaustion. He ate well of all the extra tasty bits we could gather for him and he displayed tons of guts. The amputation stump seemed to heal well and caused little pain, but the combination of so many illnesses finally proved too much. Less than a month later, he was dead. Syd and I were deeply saddened, our only comfort derived from the fact that we had at least tried to beat the odds, and that our patient had, at no stage, given up his fight to live.

THE DEATH ROLL OF the No. 5 Branch hospital in the valley continued to grow, with four or five men dying every day. Even now I can still imagine no other place more appalling than that death camp. In an endeavour to alleviate conditions there, Syd and I sent down what little food we could spare and every day two of our orderlies visited to help with dressings and other treatments. The orderlies acted under our instructions, but always in our absence — following the guards' discovery of our amputation patient, there would have been severe repercussions for all if Syd and I were ever found there again.

In our own camp, the pressure on the men to finish the Railway was intense. 'Blitz' sick parades were frequent, and even the Shomuka (camp headquarters administration clerks) were sent to work. There was a reduction in the Buppin (men allocated to perform camp and sanitation duties) and some of my orderlies were again forced to join working parties.

We soon had another two psychiatric cases, more than likely the result of cerebral malaria — a form of malignant tertian malaria which infects the brain cells causing delirium and madness. They lay on their beds with vacant gazes, alternating between periods of intense fear and milder anxiety. I remember one of the men used to stare up into the bamboo crossbeams of the hut, convinced that we needed to pull his motorbike down before it fell on him. Delusions such as these were typical. These men were well cared for by their mates. The support of a mate offered unrivalled comfort, reassuring the patient that he was not alone and helping him to bear the unbearable. The bonds of true mateship as we knew it had no limits.

The death figures of Anderson Force remained disturbing: between the middle of July (when we arrived at Mizale) and the middle of August, we lost another eight of our men from a mixture of dysentery (in the main), pellagra, malaria, beriberi, malnutrition and exhaustion, and one with cholera.[3] Five of these deaths occurred at the 55 Kilo hospital, one at the 30 Kilo hospital and the remaining two in our camps at Mizale and Apparon. It was devastating to watch men deteriorate and die in such speedy succession.

I had long been quietly considering why it was that some of our men died while others, in similar circumstances and with the same treatment, survived. My own conclusion was that some men died due to a lack of the will to live — and by that I mean a psychologically negative state — but I had also observed that many men succumbed as a result of a positive will to die. It was the equivalent of what I called 'bone pointing', with the man in question pointing the bone squarely at *himself*. I had watched semiconscious men nigh unto death for a couple of weeks, and then, as soon as their condition gradually improved and they became aware of what was going on around them, it was as if they took one look at their mates dying close by and made a definite decision: 'Oh, to hell with all this, I don't want to be here any more.' And then they would be gone — even though, medically speaking, some might have had a very good chance of recovering.

When these men were closest to death, I don't think they were strong enough to make the decision to let go, but as soon as they started to get better, it was as if they suddenly gained the strength and willpower to actively give up. I could see it in their faces. After tending to a man, often for weeks at a time, following his progress every step of the way, it was truly heartbreaking to witness him give up. Medical care can take a man to a certain point but, from what I witnessed, I came to believe a patient must possess the will to live if he had any chance of surviving.

BRIGADIER VARLEY PAID US a visit on 14 August, accompanied by Colonel Nagatomo. In his usual thorough manner, Varley inspected the camp in general and the sick in particular. He had just returned from the 105 and 108 Kilo camps and claimed that our sick were the worst along the line, probably due to the shattering demands of line laying. Thirty of our sick (twelve from Anderson Force and eighteen from Williams Force) were immediately selected to be sent to the 55 Kilo camp hospital later that day. Only days later, also thanks to the urging of Varley, three more parties of sick, 168 men in total, were also moved to the

55 Kilo camp hospital, and another 103 were due to follow soon after. There had been an alarming number of deaths in Williams Force — 70, in the previous ten weeks alone — and many more seemed likely to die at any time.

Jim Armstrong became very ill with a bout of diarrhoea that followed his last attack of malaria. With a certain amount of opposition from him, I at last managed to remove him from his duties at the hospital, which he was forbidden even to visit, and installed him in the main camp. There was just a chance that he would rest.

My own health was also deteriorating rapidly: a combination of diarrhoea, malaria, lack of sleep and periods of losing my appetite due to jaundice was definitely catching up with me. Following the camp inspection by Nagatomo and Varley, I was ordered by Nagatomo, with Varley's prompting, to take a 'holiday'. I later learned that Varley had pointed out to Nagatomo that some of the medical officers, who had been in the jungle all along, were showing signs of wear and needed recognition for their work. When big-hearted Nagatomo had generously offered a bonus of some few yen to the month's salary and a tin of condensed milk, the brigadier reportedly told him what to do with the bonus and milk and suggested that a more practical way of expressing his gratitude would be to exchange, for at least a brief period of time, the medical officers in the jungle with medical officers who had been attached to the base camps, where conditions were somewhat better.

Weeks later, I was shown a copy of the POW Standing Order 17 issued from Colonel Nagatomo's headquarters, which I recorded in my diary:

In order to alleviate temporarily the task of the Doctors who have continually worked with the utmost zeal and give them the opportunity to foster their health, there will now be a temporary change of POW doctors as mentioned below:

Major Hobbs to change with Major Krantz
Major Chalmers [to change with] Captain Richards
Captain Higgin [to change with] Captain Anderson
Captain Huls [to change with] Captain In't Veld.[4]

Having been brought up in the 1920s, at a time when showing emotion or admitting one couldn't cope were clear signs of weakness, I never would have conceded that, physically, I could not have lasted much longer. But Varley really knew his men and recognising that I was buggered, my health at that stage being well beyond poor, he had engineered a 'holiday' of sorts, to save me from myself. Varley, I suspect, saved me from being buried in the virgin jungles of Burma.

CHAPTER TWELVE

A BRIEF RESPITE
Apparon (80 Kilo camp) to Retpu Hospital (30 Kilo camp),
then to Little Nike (131 Kilo camp)
August–October 1943

Syd Krantz and I left Apparon on 30 August. While we were relieved to be granted a brief rest, we were more than apprehensive about leaving our men. We were also somewhat concerned for our replacements, Major Chalmers and Major Hobbs, who were largely unaccustomed to conditions in jungle working camps. We hoped that our men, who had always been so fiercely loyal to us, would not give them too much of a hard time.

During our journey to Retpu, Syd and I spent the night with the British No. 2 Mobile Force at the 62 Kilo camp, where we were very well treated. We were delayed there for a day owing to a rail accident in which two Japanese guards had been killed and six injured. The Japanese in the area were running around madly. I was infuriated that they could be so alarmed by a couple of deaths and a mere handful of injuries considering their gross lack of concern and respect for the deaths, casualties and illnesses of our men.

The following day, Syd and I were ordered to march, carrying all our gear, to the 60 Kilo camp, where we were picked up by a motor truck and taken to Retpu Hospital. It was a rough trip and on arrival we were stiff and sore. Such a march would not usually have troubled us, but we had lost a lot of condition, largely from having worked continual round-the-clock shifts during the cholera, malaria and dysentery epidemics, and I was also suffering from another prolonged attack of dysentery. I felt wretched.

The hospital camp featured a well-supplied canteen (hardly surprising considering how close it was to headquarters) and huts in good condition; hygiene was generally satisfactory. Because this was not a 'working' camp, the guards, most of whom were Korean, were not subjected to Japanese engineers pressuring them to provide fit workers, so the atmosphere was very relaxed in comparison to any other camp I had experienced. No bashings and no haggling over the sick: it was a different world.

My job consisted of looking after 200 convalescent medical cases, most of whom were suffering malaria, cholera and diarrhoea. I examined about fifteen to twenty new cases each day as well as being responsible for 26 of the worst dysentery cases. My daily rounds of the new cases could easily have been completed in less than 30 minutes, but I endeavoured to extend them to over about an hour and a half, so I could chat to men along the way. There were many lads in this hospital whom I had not seen since Tavoy, and although I had been loath to leave Jim Armstrong and his team at Apparon, I admit it gave me the greatest of pleasure to see and speak with old friends again.

The patients at Retpu were among the healthiest to be seen along the line. Some had been in this hospital since arriving ill in Tavoy, and had never been in a working party. The majority of patients, though, had been sent there from jungle camps and, well aware of their good fortune, they were not keen to see their position change. The most obvious difference I noticed between these patients and those along the Railway was their mood: these men had resigned themselves to not only accepting their own fate, but also making the most of it. Not living with the constant fear of brutal guards, of course, made their task far easier. They were motivated to improve their lives; some of the more enterprising patients set up coffee stalls (the 'coffee' made from burned rice) and also sold biscuits (baked with rice). Looking around me, I could not help but wonder how many other prisoners of war could have been saved had it been possible to exchange some of these men with their deathly ill comrades out in the working camps. It was a disgrace that many had been kept here for so long, but it was impossible to assess the degree of responsibility. I suspected it did not lie all with the Japanese.

My days at Retpu were restful and largely undisturbed. Reveille was at 0730 hours with breakfast half an hour later. I commenced my rounds at 1000 hours and tried to spin them out until lunchtime. By the orders of both the Japanese and our own command, Lieutenant Colonel Chris Black (the commanding officer of Black Force), we then went to our dispersal areas at 1300 hours and returned at 1615 hours. The dispersal area was anywhere within 300 metres of the camp boundary, embracing a stretch of water some 500 to 600 metres long. Within this area we were free to roam, rather like animals in a zoo enclosure. Along the banks, the men had built all sorts of shelters from bamboo and *attap*, where they retired in peace during the afternoon. The usual routine began with a swim and a wash followed by a sleep, reading or a game of chess or cards, followed by another swim before returning to camp. The weather was glorious, somewhat reminiscent of springtime back home. All in all, according to captivity standards, these afternoons left very little to be desired.

The third of September marked the fourth anniversary of the commencement of the war. With time on my hands, memories of the eve of war came flooding back to me. I remembered walking arm in arm along Manly wharf with my dear friend Barbara Blazey, sheets of newspapers flip-flapping across our paths, with no inkling of what would soon follow. I wondered if Barbie was also thinking of that night. I was in a rare, somewhat wistful mood. I couldn't help but smile when I thought about my trip to Dapto, when I took command of the Sound Ranging Group with a brand new pip on my shoulder: it had been a major milestone in my life and look where it had led me. I had no regrets. Being away from violent guards enabled my mind to unravel a little, as if a heavy cloud had lifted and, even if only for a brief time, I enjoyed indulging in my own memories.

Later that same afternoon, back in camp, I witnessed the first brilliant sunset I had seen for some months: a delightful, ever-changing combination of pink, russet, khaki and blue. It was a colour scheme I have never seen anywhere except in Burma. A concert was held in the parade ground under the full moon; the hospital had managed to retain some musicians and artists to entertain the patients. The men sat cross-legged in the dirt and waited for the entertainment, which included quality music, comedy acts and jokes: a cabaret of sorts. Even the guards attended, joining in to sing 'Auld Lang Syne'. These concerts offered all of us a chance to forget; to escape through genuine laughter and joy. I thought of the poor devils in the working camps and hoped that they, too, would again be able to enjoy such pleasures.

The combined effect of the spectacular sunset, the new moon, the concert and the memories of four years ago made me feel as though I was on the cusp of a new era. I experienced a peculiar, but pleasant, feeling of elation which is difficult to describe, even now, but it was very real at the time. It was like looking down upon my life from somewhere above, viewing it from a new angle. After only days of resting in a relatively peaceful and quiet place, away from epidemics and enjoying glorious fine days of sunshine and better food, my physical health was improving and, mentally, I was already filled with renewed hope.

IN MID–SEPTEMBER THE Japanese made a *presento* of one tin of milk per eleven men, three kilograms of margarine for sixteen men, and 40 cigars per man. This was an uncommon and unexplained act of generosity on their behalf, and with plenty of bananas and limes and some eggs already in our possession it was the most food I had seen in quite some time. I tried to imagine any of the guards in charge of Anderson Force giving us such treats, but it was incomprehensible.

With new foods available, I decided to experiment with the diet of my dysentery patients in an endeavour to control oedema and soft motions. Up until this time, the dysentery patients had been receiving a diet of a pappy, watery stew. I asked the cooks to prepare rice boiled with vegetables and meat which, when thoroughly cooked, was then placed into pans and baked in the improvised camp ovens. This food was more palatable and had far less fluid content than the patients were used to. The eggs and bananas provided by Red Cross funds were also cooked with rice to make baked custards. Almost immediately the daily average number of motions of the dysentery patients was significantly reduced.

My workload remained light in the mornings and I had plenty of time during the afternoons to rest, read, chat and play contract bridge with Syd and others. I enjoyed an interesting discussion with a Dutch doctor, Captain In't Veld, on the possible causes of central scotoma — a form of blindness which affects central vision, as opposed to peripheral vision, and a condition from which some of our men had been suffering. We debated whether it could have been due to beriberi, pellagra or if it was perhaps vascular. It was a thought-provoking chat, but largely academic as, regardless of the cause, there was nothing we could do to treat the condition. We also debated the possible causes of the higher incidence of severe tropical ulcers among the Australians at the 105 Kilo camp. The treatment adopted by the Dutch was essentially the same as we used in Anderson Force — that is, ensuring a minimal amount of trauma and *never* gouging. Not without pride, I mentioned that so far we had not yet had one amputation of any men of Anderson Force. No other force, to my knowledge, had a similar record and, in some forces the number of amputations was considerable. I counted this as one of my, and my devoted medical orderlies', most important achievements during our time on the Railway, and I remain forever grateful to my Uncle Arthur for imparting to me his knowledge and discipline which so often helped me to improvise and adapt during captivity, especially in regard to ulcers.

In such a relaxed camp, and with so much free time, it was far easier to keep my diary. In the working camps, guards frequently conducted random searches of our possessions, usually when we were moving between camps, and I was always fearful that my diary would be discovered, despite being carefully wrapped in sheets of paper at the bottom of my pack. I always took great care not only in what I wrote but also where and when I wrote. At working camps, I generally recorded my entries inside the RAP, where I also kept legitimate Japanese-approved medical records, so it did not appear particularly suspicious. Occasionally, I asked a man to keep a lookout while I wrote, just to play it safe. But in Retpu, with relatively casual guards, I was confident that an inspection was unlikely.

Books were still considered one of the greatest assets we had. I thoroughly enjoyed reading *Modern War Surgery* edited by Hamilton Bailey, a first-class publication, though largely irrelevant to my current circumstances. I was also particularly enthralled by the works of Walt Whitman, the influential American poet and writer, and John Buchan, a Scottish writer who later became governor-general of Canada. Knowing that I would soon have to trade these books to keep our mobile lending library going, I recorded a collection of quotes from the works of Whitman, Buchan and others in my diary, keen to retain a reference to their thoughts for further contemplation. It was such a luxury to have the time and space to reflect upon differing philosophies and beliefs. A couple of my favourites are:

> *The essence of civilisation lies in man's defiance of an impersonal universe.*
>
> — John Buchan

> *Everything comes out of the dirt — everything; everything comes out of the people, everyday people, the people as you find them and leave them; people, people, just people.*
>
> — Walt Whitman

The Buchan quote made me think about the dangers of apathy; and Whitman's words reminded me that whether a man was a captor or one of the captured, he was still human. At surface level, perhaps mine were simplistic observations, but at the time, I truly needed such reminders, for it was hard to accept that some of our keepers were indeed human. Both quotes also made me think about what it is that separates one human being from another. Why was it, for instance, that some guards, charged with the order to punish a prisoner of war, would beat a defenceless opponent to a bloody mess while a select few might go easy on him? Likewise, why was it that some POW officers rose to the challenge of fiercely defending their men in camps, while others reportedly accepted privileges of rank and rarely left their huts, while their own men laboured and died out on the Railway?

As far as I could see, what distinguished one human from another in captivity was his ability to make very different decisions: to accept his fate or make active judgments about the life he chose to lead, regardless of his circumstances. A prisoner of war might be treated like an animal, but he still held the power to choose not to become one, or act like one. Equally, a guard might be ordered to act like an animal, but he still held the power to choose not to become one, or at least not one so vicious. The life of a human is always filled with decisions. The ultimate challenge for us, as prisoners of war and individuals, was to search for the right kind of answers that might lead us home — with our own integrity still intact.

WE SOON LEARNED FROM Lieutenant Colonel Black that the hospital at Retpu was in the process of being disbanded and moved to the 105–130 Kilo area, closer to the working parties, and that the hospital at the 55 Kilo camp was also in the process of being moved. This meant my holiday would quickly come to an end. I was already more than grateful for the break I had received and its obvious benefits to my physical health: I had gained approximately two kilograms in one month, and felt much better for it. What's more, Syd and I had also heard rumours that the men of 'F' Force, located at a camp very close to our own men, were experiencing some form of 'horror cholera' and that their death toll was escalating. This news only made me even more anxious to return.

Much to my relief, on 8 October, I finally received orders to return to my own unit (Syd was to follow soon after). Padre Bashford, an Anglican chaplain who had at times been attached to Anderson Force, arrived at Retpu later in the day and informed us that Major Alan Hobbs, the doctor who had exchanged places with Syd Krantz, was suffering an attack of acute dysentery at the 108 Kilo camp. He also reported that one of our men, Gunner L.O.A. Smith had died of cholera at the 108 Kilo camp, and there was another suspicious case at the 131 Kilo camp. Jim Langley, the former driver of our late CO, Colonel John O'Neill, had also died. According to Padre Bashford, our men had been moved through another five camps, all of which were located in the worst cholera area: Songkurai, in Thailand. I agitated to depart immediately.

THE 'WELCOME HOME' I received from my men at Little Nike (131 Kilo camp) was a thrill I will long remember. As I climbed off the back of the truck, Jim Armstrong, John Shaw, Don Kerr, Pinkey Rhodes and many others rushed towards me, their lean arms outstretched. Relieved and grateful to be among my own, I was suddenly overcome with emotion and struggled to control a flood of tears on the brink of bursting. It was strange to think how all of us had originally been thrown together — our companionship imposed at random by our own Division Headquarters — and now, being back with my men was like returning to family. There was an unspoken affinity amongst us all; we belonged together. 'Rowley's back' spread rapidly through the camp, and more men were soon on the scene to welcome me. Colonel Williams greeted me warmly, with a handshake and a smile; even Colonel Anderson, still the perfect gentleman, acknowledged me politely with a firm handshake.

I was appalled by just how much the condition of all men had deteriorated in a six-week period. The gruelling ordeal of the previous weeks was apparent in every face throughout the camp. Nearly all had lost more weight; they looked haggard and old beyond their young years. Their skin, toasted a dirty brown from the hot sun appeared even more wrinkled. Some stared at me with seemingly unseeing eyes. I felt indescribably guilty that I had deserted my men, living the 'soft life' in Retpu when they had so obviously needed me.

On my way to my quarters, John Shaw and Don Kerr briefed me on their camp moves during my absence and then, inside the RAP, John Chalmers, Jim Armstrong and Pinkey Rhodes relayed to me the experiences of the sick. The health of the men had descended to unimaginable depths. From Apparon (80 Kilo camp), most of the men had moved on foot to Kyondaw (95 Kilo camp). John Chalmers, my replacement, had remained at the 80 Kilo camp with one of our men, Norris, who was suffering from cholera, and who later died. Days later, the men had been forced to march for nine hours to the 108 Kilo camp in Thailand, near the border. During the journey they had stopped briefly at the 105 Kilo camp for breakfast, and Major Alan Hobbs had remained there with 50 of the sickest men, including one who subsequently died of cholera. With both Chalmers and Hobbs separated from the main body of Anderson Force, the working parties were temporarily left without a doctor. Work on the Railway had continued and by the middle of September the men were moved again — the majority on foot — to the 116 Kilo camp, arguably the worst POW camp on the Railway.

In spite of the eloquence with which John Shaw and Don Kerr tried to describe this camp to me, I found it difficult to believe that man could exist in such surroundings. These camps were in the midst of the worst cholera camps previously occupied by the tragic 'F' Force. The huts where our men had been expected to sleep were situated at the foot of a gully with a stream flowing right through the centre of it. Above the camp were several huts occupied by Burmese and native Indians, many of whom were suffering from cholera and most of them from dysentery or some other bowel complaint. During this period it rained as only it can in the tropics, and the huts had been practically awash with floodwaters carrying faeces and other debris from the camps above. According to John Chalmers, it had been impossible to keep one's feet dry, with the floors of the huts under some 30 to 40 centimetres of mud, slush and human faeces.

After four days at this dire camp, the men had received orders to move to the 122 Kilo camp (near Songkurai, in Thailand). A group of 200 of the sick were returned to the 105 Kilo camp, where Alan Hobbs remained, leaving only 600 in the combined Anderson and Williams Forces. In those camps over 800 men of 'F' Force had died, most of them from cholera, and still more continued to die each day. A week later, Anderson and Williams Forces — also joined by 300 Dutch — moved to Little Nike (131 Kilo camp), with the majority of men forced to march nine kilometres in spite of the fact that rail had been laid right to the camp. Colonel Williams, once more standing up for his men, received a brutal bashing courtesy of a rifle butt and the boot of a guard. Since arriving at Little Nike one of our men had died of cholera and two others from a combination of dysentery, fatigue and general exhaustion.

It was devastating to listen to these men recount their recent journeys. In every respect their experiences at these camps had surpassed — by far — anything I had lived through on the Railway, particularly from the point of view of incessant work, poor food, low morale and so-called 'living' quarters. Twelve men from Anderson Force had died while I was away.

Back with my men, there was a lot of work to be done. The hospital patients were all very ill, and every day more and more men collapsed while out at work and needed to be admitted to hospital. Jim Armstrong was again stricken with diarrhoea; he had lost considerable weight in my absence. The mental and physical strain of the previous weeks had taken a heavy toll on my friend and I was desperate to see him rest. Don Kerr continued to do a magnificent job in carrying out the administration of the camp. I hated to think what would have become of Anderson Force if we ever lost him. His administrative ability was something that had to be seen at close quarters to be appreciated. Without him, my job — and that of John Chalmers during my absence — would have been almost impossible. He knew every man in the force and, despite being medically unqualified, he could assess the physical condition and capabilities of each man nearly as well as we could.

With the two ends of the Railway soon due to be joined, the engineers became even more unforgiving in their *speedo! speedo!* campaigns. All men, apart from hospital cases, were sent to work, forced to labour in stretches of 24 to 32 hours at a time, with only a few hours in camp to recuperate before being sent out again. Despite their utter exhaustion, in the lead-up to the 'big day' there was a general mood of relief among our men in camp. Eternal optimists, most were hopeful that, following the completion of such a monumental Nippon achievement, there might be a period of rest in store as a reward for their hard work. They clung to the hope that, with the Railway complete, the life of a prisoner of war might just become, at the very least, a little bit easier.

IT WAS MID-OCTOBER, and on the day before the two ends of the Railway were joined all men were sent to work for 36 to 48 hours straight. There was little opportunity for me to negotiate on behalf of the sick: the guards, frenetic to see the culmination of their achievement, were determined to send any skeleton that could still walk out to work. Only the bedridden remained in camp.

During the day, while I was tending to the sick, the guards advised that there was a 'very special job' that needed to be done, and I was ordered to provide more men for this unspecified mission. The guards made it clear that there would be no value in me resisting their orders on this day and so I was forced to select about six of the least sick men in camp — most of whom were suffering malaria, dysentery, malnutrition and exhaustion. As it turned out, these men were detailed to convert tree trunks into square totem poles using adzes and axes which, when inscribed with apparently appropriate Japanese hieroglyphics, were to become memorials to the POWs who held 'the honour' of losing their lives during the course of the construction of the Railway.

The Railway was finally joined somewhere around the 145 Kilo mark on 17 October:[1] a cause of great rejoicing among the guards and engineers. I was in camp with the sick when the 'festivities' commenced, but the men relayed events to me upon their return. They told me that Japanese high officials had travelled from all over to be present at the great ceremony, arriving in open steel rail trucks which, to mark the occasion, had been transformed by the addition of tiny *attap* roofs precariously perched on thin bamboo poles. From what I heard, no Egyptian king could have believed he was travelling with greater pomp and ceremony; such were their delusions of grandeur.

While the Japanese celebrated their feat of engineering brilliance, one that would make their beloved Emperor eternally proud, exhausted, disease-ravaged and starving prisoners of war thought of their fallen mates. Among the dead and dying along the Railway were at least 2815 Australians,[2] men whose lives had been so unnecessarily wasted at the hands of our degenerate keepers, and all in a pathetic cause.

CHAPTER THIRTEEN

NEW JOURNEYS
Little Nike (131 Kilo camp), to Tamarkan, Thailand
October 1943–February 1944

The very morning after the Railway was joined, working parties were ordered to carry out repairs and maintenance. Any hope we'd had of the men being granted a reprieve from slave labour now seemed fanciful.

Not long after the men had left for work, Syd Krantz returned to our camp, replacing John Chalmers, who was to be transferred to the 55 Kilo camp. I wasted no time filling Syd in on events that had taken place in our absence, just as they had been relayed to me by John Shaw, John Chalmers, Don Kerr, Jim and Pinkey more than a week ago. His reaction was similar to mine: guilt, incredulity and an immediate need to help. From the bottom of his pack Syd produced a wad of Thai money, sent for us by Don Murchison, the International Red Cross representative. Pennies from heaven, so to speak. Since crossing the border into Thailand, our Burmese currency had become worthless and, despite perpetual promises from the Japanese that we would soon be paid in Thai rupees, they continued to pay us in Burmese currency. We had been living in a new land without any access to cash to trade with locals, something which was essential for subsidising our meagre rations.

Armed with the cash, I left Syd and collected Jim Armstrong from the RAP, telling him we were going on a journey. (Ordering Jim on a mission was one of the only ways to force him to take a break from his duties.) We both changed into our 'Sunday best': well-worn shorts, shirt and a slouch hat. We were hardly starched and pressed, but as a matter of pride, many of us saved our only 'best outfit' for whenever we were allowed to travel outside of camp. We wanted to present the best possible front: we were soldiers still.

With Sergeant Shimojo's permission, our guard led the way, his loaded rifle by his side. We marched through the jungle until we reached the edge of a river which we would have to wade through to reach the village of Nike on the other side. We watched as our guard stripped off down to his G-string, neatly folded his clothes and rested them on top of his head. He then made his way across, the water level rising almost up to his armpits, his rifle raised towards the sun. We followed behind, the water level only reaching up to our hips. Jim and I were both amused and impressed by our guard's problem-solving technique — without doubt, one of the only genuine displays of 'guard logic' we had witnessed. Reaching the far bank, the guard bathed himself, dried off with his tightly wrung G-string, dressed and then ordered us to proceed to the village.

I was glad to have the opportunity to speak with Jim alone, to discuss privately how his health really was and how he and the other orderlies had coped in my absence. The formerly big man was now a gaunt figure, but Jim Armstrong was never a man to complain; he always maintained the face of an optimist. We chatted quietly to each other all the way to Nike, old friends reunited, trailing behind our uninterested guard.

Walking along the main road of Nike, Jim and I could not help but stare at the locals — most of whom were dressed in Western-style clothing. After living in the jungle for so long it seemed beyond belief that we were now strolling through a relatively sophisticated village. We had re-entered civilisation, where people operated shops and markets, drove elephants and were policed by men in gold-braided uniforms.

Our guard disappeared into a shop, leaving us to trade with locals. We spent most of Syd's money on milk and bananas. I attempted to bargain with my Burmese rupees, but to no avail. However, when the locals realised that our purchases were for the sick, they generously gave us some sago flour and *goula malacca* (tasty, sweet sugar from palm). They told us they had heard of the terrible fate of prisoners of war suffering cholera in the Nike and Three Pagodas Pass area, especially near Songkurai, and offered their sympathy through kind words and generosity.

As Jim and I followed our guard out of Nike, we took a long look at our surroundings. There was so much food in this village and it made us seethe with resentment when we thought of how many more lives could have been saved had we received our pay in local currency upon arrival in Thailand.

ALL RAILWAY WORK CEASED, temporarily, on 19 October. I was given a party of 50 men, under Lieutenant John Ross (of the 2/15th Field Regiment), in an endeavour to clean the camp area in general and the river area in particular. We had heard rumours that Nagatomo would soon be visiting our camp on his way through to Burma and suspected our guards were anxious to get the place into a presentable state.

A week later, Colonel Nagatomo, accompanied by Colonel Nakamura, a senior Japanese commander in Thailand, arrived to inspect our camp. Our guards must have received either high praise or a terrific blitzing, because following the departure of the colonels they were all rotten drunk. For the next 24 hours there was not one guard on duty. Stuck in the middle of the jungle, we had nowhere to run, but appreciated a reprieve from their presence, especially their big sticks.

The visit from Nagatomo and Nakamura was enough to kick-start a new wave of speculation about our post-Railway future. The men thrived on rumours (or, as they were affectionately known, 'latrine furphies' because new theories were usually spread from one man to another while visiting the latrine). Everyone wanted to believe that a new and better life lay somewhere ahead. Various scenarios flashed around camp at lightning speed: Bangkok, Singapore and Saigon (present-day Ho Chi Minh City) were all cited as possible destinations; as well as the less exciting option of the 116 Kilo camp, where we might be forced to carry out never-ending rail maintenance work. Our hopes were raised by our observation that the Japanese were becoming very edgy, possibly at the prospect of further Allied bombings. Evidence of their growing paranoia was the fact that they now refused to allow us to gather in groups larger than three or four, fearing attacks of violence from prisoners of war. (Imagine — from unarmed, sick and starving men!)

By the end of the month the wet season had passed, leaving more dead men in its wake. As of 31 October 1943, we had lost a total of 69 out of 739 men from Anderson Force (9.3 per cent) along the Railway.[1] Cerebral malaria also continued to ravage our men. Often beginning as a seemingly ordinary case of malaria, after three to six days the patient became delirious, combative and difficult to control. After a further two to three days, he became exhausted and semi-comatose, and when the original attack of malaria subsided, continuous fever followed, but without the customary rigors or sweating. The semi-comatose period usually lasted from two to four days, and then there was either a very gradual recovery or, more frequently, the patient became unconscious and developed rapid, gasping respirations, then slowly quietened and died. Intravenous quinine and M&B 693, one of the first anti-bacterial sulphur drugs, were tried in varying doses but without any dramatic beneficial results. Some cases, before developing fever, showed signs of weakness in the legs and a few collapsed while seemingly quite fit. These patients required round-the-clock nursing by the dedicated orderlies.

One night a Dutch lad suffering from cerebral malaria fled from his hospital bed, terrified by delusions that he was about to be shot. He lumbered off into the darkness clad only in a shirt. When his absence was noted by the night medical orderly, we immediately informed the Japanese, who then called a *tenko* at 0300 hours. Search parties of POWs were at once sent out, accompanied by a Korean guard. We searched for hours on end in the darkness, without any luck. It was not until after 1000 hours the next morning that he was found on a hill just above the camp, much to the relief of everyone, including the Japanese. He was brought back to the camp and put into hospital again, not much the worse for wear. The guards, realising the boy was mentally deranged — and probably relieved at not having to report an escape to their headquarters — inflicted no punishment on the patient, orderlies or staff. Not immediately anyway.

Following this incident, we were ordered to mount our own guard, one at each end of our hospital hut, every night to keep a lookout for deluded patients attempting escape. A few nights later, The Storm Trooper, the barbaric Korean guard, checked the hospital hut at the watch changeover time, only to discover that one of our men was not yet at his post. He pulled Colonel Anderson and Bill Drower from their beds, as well as the off-duty guard, Sergeant Lynch, and his relief, Sergeant Maher. Their punishment was brutal. By the time the four men were brought to me in the RAP they were in a very bad way. Having only just regained consciousness, their eyes were glazed. They were beaten black and blue, with bruising, bleeding, contusions and lacerations to their faces and heads. Colonel Anderson had an egg-sized lump on his head.

As I cleaned and dressed my CO's messy wounds, I felt the stirring of a new understanding for this man with whom I had long been at odds. Throughout my 'holiday' at Retpu, with so much time to reflect, I had gradually come to recognise that every individual can possess differing views and beliefs, religious or otherwise, which then lead him to take very different actions. One man's action in any given situation will nearly always be judged by at least some observers to be correct, while others, especially if they possess differing beliefs, might protest vehemently. In such a scenario, objectively, who is right? I had begun to question how any man — especially me — could criticise the actions of another if he had never been in *exactly* the same circumstances. After all, I had never been the CO of Anderson Force. How could I really know what Anderson was experiencing and therefore basing his own decisions upon? I vowed to try to be more tolerant.

ONE HUNDRED MEN WERE sent out to the Railway to perform so-called 'light work' on 9 November, but thankfully returned to camp the following afternoon. Apart from those on essential duties, all men were, at long last, allowed to rest for a few days. I took the opportunity to tend to a matter that had long been worrying me. In addition to my diary, I had been writing personal letters as well as preparing weekly medical reports on sickness rates and food. The bulk of paper I was carrying was becoming more and more of an embarrassment, and I was growing nervous that the guards might soon become suspicious.

Late one night, inside the RAP, with my faithful orderlies on watch, I sat at a small bamboo table and began summarising Part 1 of my diary, as well as my records of illnesses and rations. Using a fountain pen I had purchased from one of my men for seven rupees back at Taunzan, I squeezed as many words as I could onto each page. I ended up with a condensed version of Part 1 of my diary plus a single table listing the records of illnesses and rations. In all, it ran to seven and a half pages. It took me several nights but when completed, I secreted the summary amongst my legitimate medical records for safekeeping. I remember looking at my pile of original papers, knowing that with the summary now taken care of I really should destroy them. But I couldn't, they were like old friends by then. Throwing caution to the wind, I hid Part 1 of my original diary in the bottom of my pack and then tucked my letters home next to my summary inside my medical records.

On 20 November, Colonel Nagatomo ordered all camps to hold another special memorial service in honour of men who had lost their lives on the Railway. Elaborate crosses, hand-carved at our own headquarters, were sent to POW camps especially for the occasion. We gathered in the cemetery standing to attention, each man dressed smartly and proudly in his best rags. Colonel Anderson delivered the opening address and one of the padres conducted the service. As wreaths made from wild flowers and leaves were placed on the graves, I wondered how many more memorial services we would have to endure before being released.

Sergeant Shimojo read a speech from Colonel Nagatomo in honour of the deceased prisoners of war. It was maddening to have to endure such heartfelt hypocrisy:

This tragedy [deaths on the Railway] is a result of the war, however, it is owing to fate that you are in this condition, and I consider that God has called you here.[2]

It might have been war that brought us to the Railway, but neither God nor fate had called our mates to their graves. The Japanese were entirely responsible for their deaths.

OUR CAMP CONTINUED TO hum with rumours. The 1000 sickest men from the recently combined forces of No. 3 Branch (to which Anderson Force belonged) and No. 5 Branch Thai POW camps were said to be heading to a new hospital in a camp near Bangkok; 6500 others bound for a 'rest' camp; with maintenance parties of 3000 to be left along the Railway line.

I spent little time worrying about where we were headed next; I was too busy trying to keep our sick men alive. By the end of November, the sick figures were still increasing, with only 35 men of Anderson Force working. Since the middle of the month, we had received no meat, just peas and beans with occasional pumpkin, sweet potatoes and melons to colour our watery stew. There were a few cases of beriberi and pellagra and some of the ulcer cases were also becoming worse. Four more of our men died, including Sergeant Lynch, who after recovering from his severe bashing by The Storm Trooper had experienced an attack of cerebral malaria and then, a week later, succumbed to yet another recurrence of malaria.

By now, I, too, was again stricken with malaria. Earlier in the month, the Japanese had conducted blood examinations of the camp and reported that Syd Krantz had benign tertian malaria and I had subtertian malaria (two different strains). Aside from lassitude and weakness, I wasn't suffering any other symptoms. Malaria, in all its incarnations, never ceased to confound me. An extensive variety of symptoms could accompany this disease, including high fever, sweating, rigors, a rash around the mouth, severe headaches — even blackwater fever, where the kidneys become damaged and blood is present in a patient's urine. As we moved from camp to camp, I could tell if the men were being infected by a new strain because the symptom patterns would change. In one area there would be a predominance of headaches, in another, perhaps muscle pain. If we spent an extended period of time at a particular camp, we could sometimes build up immunity to whatever strain of malaria was present, but as soon as we moved to another camp we were immediately vulnerable to a new strain.

Malaria, like violence, was virtually impossible to escape.

BY ORDERS OF JAPANESE headquarters, I was included in an advance party of 50 men to be sent from Anderson Force, under Major Don Kerr and Major Rupert Barraclough, to take over the camp at Tamarkan (about 55 kilometres north of Non Pladuk[3] in Thailand) for No. 3 Branch and No. 5 Branch personnel. No reason was given but we suspected ongoing Railway maintenance work was in store. We had heard that Tamarkan, under the command of outstanding British senior officer Colonel Toosey, was one of the best-run camps in Thailand. For once it seemed likely that our next camp would be better than the last.

Our advance party moved from Little Nike on 12 December and spent the night at Kanchanaburi, more commonly known as Kanburi, near the site of the so-called 'Bridge Over the River Kwai' — later to be made famous by the novel and film of the same name. We travelled to Tamarkan, some four kilometres north-west of the township of Kanchanaburi, the following day.

Upon arrival at Tamarkan, we were thoroughly searched by guards and I lost Part 1 of my diary. It wasn't the frightening ordeal I had long anticipated. The guard simply plucked my papers from the bottom of my pack and tossed them aside without comment. Having been briefed to search for illicit radio parts, the guard wasn't even vaguely interested in the contents of my carefully wrapped notebook. Had he been ordered to search for diaries, I might not have been so lucky: such was the random and illogical nature of camp searches. The guard failed to notice the second part of my diary, my letters home and my summary — all of which were still secreted in amongst my official medical records. I was very disappointed to have lost the first part of my diary, but not devastated; after all, I still had a summary of Part 1 and I had escaped punishment. In light of what could have happened, I counted my blessings.

Following the search, we were welcomed by the rear party of Colonel Toosey's camp (Colonel Toosey and the main body of troops had already left). The personnel were mainly British with a few Australians and their generosity and kindness was more than we could possibly have hoped for. We were given a feed — and I mean a *real* feed. The men were taken over by the ORs (other ranks, other than officers) and given so much to eat that food had actually to be returned to the kitchen! Along with Don and Rupert, I was taken to the officers' mess where we enjoyed meat, vegetables, eggs — and even savouries and cakes (made from rice) from the canteen.

The first of the main body from the 55 Kilo hospital arrived with Colonel Albert 'Bertie' Coates around Christmas time.[4] Coates was now the senior medical officer of the No. 3 and No. 5 Branches at Tamarkan, including the hospital, while Colonel Ramsay (commanding officer of Ramsay Force) was the CO of the entire camp.

Our food continued to improve and was maintained at a fairly constant level: 150 grams of meat, 500–600 grams of vegetables, 600 grams of rice, plus oil and salt, per man per day. The canteen service was adequate, there being an ample and constant supply of eggs and bananas, with occasional pawpaws and limes — as well as precious cigarettes and tobacco.

Smoking had long been a problem much-maligned by medical staff. Some of our blokes had, in the past, sold their rations for a cigarette; they were more hungry for a smoke than a feed. In some of the camps, we had to bring these men outside the officers' mess, put them on parade and then order them to sit down and eat their rations (actually standing over them to make sure they did). We soon discovered that several of these men had pre-sold their meal for cigarettes they had already smoked, so the men expecting extra rice were not happy with our intervention. At least in Tamarkan the men could enjoy a smoke without forgoing a meal.

I remained RMO of Anderson Force, but was also given the official job of hygiene medical officer of the combined No. 3 and No. 5 Branches. As adjutant (a role invented for me by Coates) I became the 'go-between' for Coates and the casualty clearing station officers, who took control over the administration of the hospital. I carried out my new role in conjunction with Major Colin Cameron of Western Australia, the hygiene officer, and between us, and with the assistance of Don Kerr, we took over the management of all essential services: the kitchens, the laundry, the sanitation services, gardens, cattle yards, duck yards, pig pens, canteen services, sports and concert parties. The camp was run almost along the lines of peacetime barracks. It seemed we had escaped the jungle and arrived in the Garden of Eden.

TOWARDS THE END OF February, a flood of troops streamed from the jungle into our camp. Something was definitely up, but before our own rumours had time to swirl, the Japanese announced that 900 men were to be selected for the 'Japan Party'. Mission, as usual, not stated. The party was to be divided into six *kumis* each of 150 men, plus one officer of less than field rank in charge and one Australian Army Medical Corps personnel as medical support. Work parties were usually selected by our own officers — as had been the case with 'A' Force — but this time we would have very little say, and certainly there would be no opportunity to keep any of our military units intact.

Early one morning all prisoners at Tamarkan were ordered on parade to be inspected by Japanese medical officers. As they walked up and down the long lines of men, it was immediately apparent that the Japanese were only interested in the younger and fitter of us. The eyes of the medical inspectors quickly passed over any man with greying hair or any obvious injuries or signs of physical weakness. By the end of that same day, the Japanese had compiled their list of 900 names, but it wasn't until March that the party would be finalised. There were assorted feelings amongst our men about the prospect of selection. Some thought life in Japan — away from tropical diseases, low-rank guards and the possibility of an Allied attack at Tamarkan — would have to be better; surely it couldn't be any worse than Railway life? Others, though, me included, contemplated the risk of being torpedoed by an Allied submarine during a sea voyage to Japan.

When the list was finally made public to us, my name was on it: RMO of Kumi No. 35. I accepted my fate; there was no other choice, but of the utmost concern to all men was being separated from his mates. I was very sad to be leaving behind Jim Armstrong, Pinkey Rhodes, Don Booth, Don Kerr and John Shaw. It was terrible trying to imagine my life ahead without them; I would be the only pea missing from our little pod.

In camp, many of the men offered me their best wishes, handshake after handshake — even Colonel Anderson — it seemed both of us had put the past behind us. But in my own group of mates, few words were spoken about my impending departure; we carried on much the same as we always had. Each of us understood what the other was feeling; it was enough just to enjoy our last days in one another's company.

On the night before I was due to depart, I asked John Shaw if he would join me for a quiet word in the RAP. John was a man I respected and admired above all others: I would carry with me his wisdom, philosophies and teachings for the rest of my life. I knew just how much he treasured his own writings and I could think of no other man I could trust more to take care of mine. It would be far too dangerous to attempt to take my writings and Part 2 of my diary on a journey to Japan, where searches would no doubt be both frequent and thorough. I had tempted fate once and escaped, but I was not confident I would be so lucky again.

Inside the RAP, John and I stood opposite one another, each of us wondering if we might ever see each other again. I fetched the bundle of letters I had written to my parents and my precious notebook.

'Would you mind delivering these to my parents,' I asked, holding my papers out towards him, 'if you should happen to beat me home.'

John nodded. He knew exactly what I meant. I knew he would. We had shared everything together, from a tiny tin of oatmeal to all our hopes and desires for a better life after the war. I had been a loner through most of my life, at ease with plenty of acquaintances but with very few close friends. I knew John Shaw was the truest friend I could ever hope for.

'Of course,' he said, stepping forward to accept my bundle. 'No trouble. No trouble at all.'

I pushed my glasses further back on the bridge of my nose to stare solidly at my friend. He had the eyes of an engineer and the mind of a poet.

'Good luck,' I offered.

'See you at home, Rowley,' he said, shaking my hand firmly.

'Yes,' I said, my lips parting into a slow smile. 'I suppose you will.'

No more words were needed.

PART FOUR

THE JAPAN PARTY

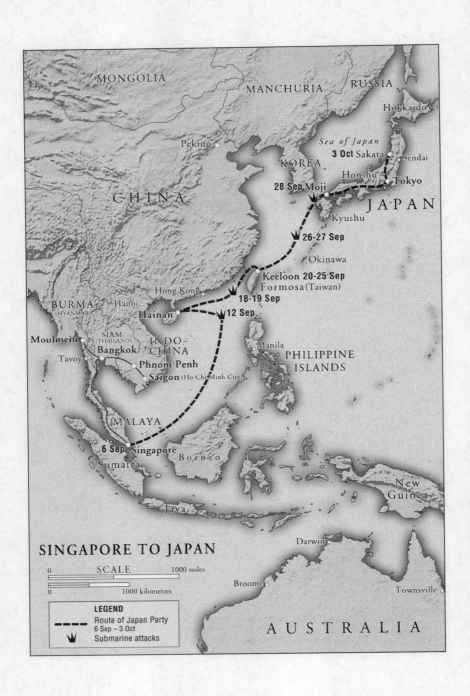

MONGOLIA

MANCHURIA

RUSSIA

Hokkaido

Peking

Sea of Japan

3 Oct Sakata

Sendai

KOREA

28 Sep Moji

Honshu

CHINA

Tokyo

JAPAN

Kyushu

26-27 Sep

Okinawa

Keelóon 20-25 Sep

Formosa (Taiwan)

Hong Kong

18-19 Sep

Hanoi

BURMA

(MYANMAR)

Hainan

12 Sep

Moulmein

SIAM

(THAILAND)

Bangkok

INDO-

CHINA

Manila

PHILIPPINE

ISLANDS

Tavoy

Phnom Penh

Saigon (Ho Chi Minh City)

MALAYA

6 Sep Singapore

Borneo

Sumatra

New

Guinea

Java

SINGAPORE TO JAPAN

Darwin

0   SCALE   1000 miles

0   1000 kilometres

Broome

Townsville

AUSTRALIA

LEGEND

- - - Route of Japan Party
6 Sep – 3 Oct

Submarine attacks

CHAPTER FOURTEEN

BURIED TREASURE
Tamarkan to Jeep Island
March–August, 1944

On 27 March, those of us selected for the Japan Party stood on parade fully clad in a brand new kit: shorts, shirt, boots, even underpants. The Japanese had issued each of us with captured AIF clothing; even our keepers realised it probably wouldn't be appropriate for us to be seen travelling in our G-strings, clogs and slouch hats. The feel of soft, clean army cloth against my skin was unfamiliar. For most of us, the clothes were far too big for our bony frames, but it was still wonderful to be in a new uniform again.

Standing on parade for hours, rows and rows of 'Nippon's chosen', we were forced to listen to a speech from a Japanese commander, a squat, podgy man bursting with self-importance. He described Japan as the 'land of milk and honey', a place of 'peace and tranquillity'. He droned on like a fire-and-brimstone preacher, full of threats and promises: 'It is a sin to eat and not work,' he said. I wondered if he'd given any thought to his own sins and if we'd still be standing on parade listening to his drivel come nightfall.

When the commander finally drew the curtain on his own smug soliloquy, it was time to wave goodbye to the mates we were forced to leave behind. All the men remaining at Tamarkan lined the road from camp to the main gates, as if forming a guard of honour at a funeral procession. As I marched away from camp, I acknowledged Jim, John, Pinkey, Don Booth and Don Kerr with a wave and a fleeting glance. 'Cheerio,' I mouthed, all I could manage, and then I quickly turned away. I had to rule a line in the ledger, at least for the time being, close off thoughts of everyone I was leaving behind and commit myself to just keeping on keeping on. If I chose to accept disappointment or defeat, I would be signing my own death warrant.

As I neared the gates of our camp, I felt a hand on my shoulder. I expected a guard, but when I turned my head, there behind me was the gentle and ever-faithful Jim Armstrong — Old Silver. Marching alongside me, he took my hand and placed something inside it. 'I want you to keep this,' he said. It was his watch, silver with a well-worn leather strap. He had been with me in the RAP only days ago when my own watch had given up the ghost. 'You'll need it more than I will,' he said. Smiling warmly, he lightly squeezed my shoulder and then made his way back to the guard of honour. I couldn't speak; it was too much, far too much. My eyes dampened as I fastened the watch to my wrist.

AFTER LEAVING TAMARKAN WE were ordered to wait in a large camp in Non Pladuk for several days so that other Japan Party *kumis* could join us. There were several 'Japan Parties' being formed from the various POW groups in Thailand: my *kumi*, No. 35, was commanded by Captain Arthur Sumner, with Warrant Officer (WO) Keith Martin as 2 i/c. Sumner, an Australian infantry company commander, was a popular choice with all the men. Kumi No. 36, marching with us, was commanded by Lieutenant Les Stupart (an old friend from Anderson Force) with WO Smith as his 2 i/c, and Corporal Len Coon as medical orderly. Kumi Nos 37, 38, 39 and 40 were due to follow shortly.

On April Fool's Day, most appropriately, we were loaded like bags of rice into enclosed steel wagons, drawn by a steam engine. There was a single sliding door in the centre of each wagon, and men jostled for a position near the opening. It was the only time there had ever been an incentive to be situated near our guards, who of course ensured they had not only the best seat in the house but also enough room to lie outstretched. There was no space for the rest of us to move; 30 to 40 men in each wagon sat with their knees beneath their chins. Inside, the air was heavy, making it difficult to breathe. Our new kit already stank of sweat. We could have fried an egg on the sides of those trucks (if only we'd had an egg!).

Every man was already exhausted and, as usual, hungry and thirsty. All we had been given to eat at the beginning of the journey was a single dixie of rice per person. Each man had had to decide for himself how best to make his ration last. Should he enjoy it all in one hit, as a complete meal while it was still fresh, or eat only a little at a time, spinning it out so there was always another spoonful, albeit stale, to look forward to? It was an impossible task considering we had no idea how long we would have to wait before receiving our next meal.

Despite only the 'fit' having been selected for the Japan Party, there was no shortage of sick for me to attend to, most of them suffering from malaria and dysentery. With no latrine facilities (not even a bucket), we were forced to take turns holding men while they hung their backsides outside the door of the moving wagon to relieve themselves. A humiliating memory, even now.

At no point during the journey were we allowed to detrain to stretch our legs and get some fresh air, not even when the train stopped at Bangkok for three hours. We just had to wait it out, trapped inside the poorly ventilated ovens until we finally arrived at Phnom Penh the following evening. I remember that night clearly: released from the wagons at last, we slept outside, stretched out under the stars. I had never been so pleased to see the sky.

The rest of our journey was in stark contrast with our rail wagon experience. The following morning we boarded a little modern steamer that carried us down the Mekong River. Up on deck, beneath the brilliance of the morning sun, I enjoyed a fleeting sensation of peace. Our day-to-day existence was a curiosity: never knowing what might come next, we always had to make the most of each good moment, and this was certainly one of them. How wonderful it was to be cruising on the swirling brown waters of one of the longest rivers in the world, surrounded by muddy shores holding back the tangled vegetation of the jungle. The guards seemed to enjoy our river cruise as much as we did, so relaxed that they were unconcerned by many of our boys singing and carrying on, all the way to Saigon.

SAIGON'S WATERFRONT WAS BUSTLING: men scurried up and down the docks like worker ants. We were now indeed a long way from the jungle. Upon arrival the guards informed us that Saigon would be our port of embarkation for Japan as soon as our ship was ready — whenever that might be. I only hoped our means of transportation to the 'land of milk and honey' would be as modern and comfortable as our lovely Mekong River steamer.

We were marched to a camp a few hundred metres past the docks. Occupied since the middle of 1942 by a party of British POWs attached to No. 1 Thai POW camp, our new home featured well-built, waterproof huts and clean grounds. Illuminated by electric lights it was as good as Hollywood to us. I could even hear music floating through the air, an orchestra rehearsing!

I was thrilled to be welcomed by a familiar face: Jim McQuillan, a British RMO I had met some time back at Nee

Soon, our first camp in Singapore. He greeted me like an old friend.

'Rowley, old chap. What a delight!' Looking me up and down without subtlety, he seemed a little taken a back by my physical appearance. 'You look as though you could do with a feed,' he said, and led the way towards the officers' mess.

Inside the mess, my eyes had to adjust to the brightness of electric lights. Boasting real tables and cane lounge chairs, it was something special. Jim kindly offered me a pewter mug filled with hot sweetened tea and we were soon joined by others, including Major John Chalmers — the base camp surgeon who had relieved me while I 'holidayed' at Retpu. I enjoyed their cheerful company and ate extraordinarily well. I hoped this might be the beginning of a new way of life.

The men were forced to return to labour, but work on the docks was almost a delight in comparison to the Railway, and it gave them ample opportunity to swipe goods and trade with the locals. Ordered to unload goods from barges to the docks, the men became proficient at springing open their crates as they passed through the shadowy area of the godown where they would quickly plant a few tins behind large cargo containers and then return to collect their heist at the end of their shift. They knocked off bolts of silk, tins of canned meat and vegetables and anything else they could get away with. The guards here were very different too: away from the pressure of the Railway and under the command of Lieutenant Yamada — in our eyes, the very best of a very bad lot from the Railway — they were far more at ease. Some of them were almost good natured, or at least far more tolerant than any others we had known.

Life in Saigon was marvellous for the health of the men. Most regained weight quite quickly and, despite a sickness rate of about 30 to 40 per cent, there were no deaths. The food was so much better than any we had eaten before and we were able to purchase eggs, bread, meat, vegetables, biscuits, fruit and even cakes from the canteen. We ate fruit salads made from pineapples, bananas and pawpaws daily, over which we poured cream made of well-beaten eggs and sugar. Saigon was paradise.

Not long into our time at Saigon, a group of British officers approached us Australian officers. They had a complaint. Some of our men had been spreading 'outlandish lies' about their experiences on the Railway, they told us, and this was disrupting the British officers' otherwise good relationships with Japanese guards. 'Please order your men to desist,' I recall one of them saying.

The British officers simply could not begin to grasp what it was like to live in the mud and slush of the wet season, or to endure the violence of the guards. They didn't believe that the Japanese failed to provide food and medicine (of which there had been plenty in Saigon). They had no idea of the killer cycle of malaria, dysentery and beriberi, the horrors of tropical ulcers and the massive death toll cholera. And how could we begin to explain?

I believe now that it was this moment that shaped my approach to talking about any of my own experiences after the war. If fellow prisoners of war could not comprehend what we had lived through, how would anyone at home have any chance of understanding? My shutters came down and I resolved that when I returned to Australia, I wouldn't try to describe, in specific terms, the enormity of our experiences.

I kept my promise for a very long time. Even now, telling my own version of events almost 60 years after the end of the war, my words will never be adequate. Unless you have supped from the same cup, you cannot know the taste.[1]

AFTER TWO ABORTIVE ATTEMPTS to embark for Japan, owing to several Allied submarines in the vicinity, the Japanese decided that the waters around Saigon were too dangerous. On 22 June, we were ordered to journey back to Phnom Penh and then to Singapore. None of us was sorry to hear this news; we were thankful to be remaining on land for the time being.

Days later, when we departed Phnom Penh for Singapore, all men marched with a precision that would have done credit to any unit. The white French population turned out in force to wave us goodbye and were obviously moved when the boys whistled 'Mademoiselle from Armentières' and 'La Marseillaise'. The French were very keen on the 'V for Victory' sign, and they went to extraordinary lengths to display it. One gentleman returned my own discreet signal in the most original exhibit possible. Dressed in his pyjamas, he was carrying out his 'daily dozen' (exercises) when he suddenly threw his body into a handstand and then slowly spread his legs, like scissor blades, into a very wide but unmistakeable 'V'. It buoyed my spirits tremendously. Such displays of support and kindness were living proof that others knew of our existence, and, what was more, they still cared.

The trip to Singapore was bloody awful. Once again we were packed into enclosed steel sweat boxes, cooped up like circus animals in transit, with 32 men per small wagon and 66 to 70 in a large wagon; there was even less room to squat than last time. Not long into the journey Sergeant Peter Britz (of the 2/15th Field Regiment) developed pneumonia. It was difficult to nurse him under such unhygienic conditions, and our guards were not willing to sacrifice any of their own carriage territory to allow him to stretch out. I still had a final few M&B 693 tablets in my personal kit, which I administered to him. He was a determined patient; I knew he would not give up — and he didn't.[2]

It was unsettling to return to Singapore Island; it was a bitter reminder of 15 February 1942 — our final day as soldiers in combat and our first as prisoners of war. I thought back to my visit to the Goodward Park Hotel, towards the end of the Malayan campaign, and remembered the grog flowing and the English men and women in their very formal and stylish attire. Now Singapore was just another devastated Japanese ghetto.

THE ATMOSPHERE ON 'JEEP ISLAND', our new home in Singapore, was tense. After spending a few days at barracks located at the River Valley Road Camp — where the food had been woefully poor, even by Railway ration standards — a party of about 150 Australian POWs were sent to construct a dry dock at the end of Jurong Road, at the south-west tip of the island of Singapore. Our new camp was on a small island, Pulau Damarlaut, about one mile distant from the worksite and under the cruel command of a Korean first class private.

Our new commander was built like a brick and we nicknamed him 'The Jeep'. He relished his power over a small bunch of Korean guards and our now very sorry-looking working party — all the men had lost the condition they had regained in Saigon. His 2 i/c was a squirt of a man we called 'Greenpants', because he wore a pair of enormous bright green trousers that swam on his puny physique. The previous experience of these two had been confined to guarding small working parties on the Railway and both were enamoured of their recent elevation in status. They were also thrilled to be in charge at such a remote location, out of reach of Lieutenant Naito, Sergeant Shimojo and all other Japanese officers who had treated them almost as badly as they had treated us.

It was comical to watch them at work, trying their utmost to mimic the behaviour of their own Japanese keepers. The Jeep seemed happiest sitting in state in the *attap*-and-bamboo guardhouse, issuing orders for food, drink and more workers, and awarding punishment at his whim. Neither The Jeep nor Greenpants seemed to have any idea of what he was really supposed to be doing and, perhaps to mask their own fears of inadequacy, they became more beastly towards us as each day passed.

By early August, pressure to complete building the dock had increased. With so many Japanese ships now lost to Allied submarines, the Japanese sent word that it was time for another *speedo! speedo!* campaign. The engineers responsible for the construction of the dock ordered The Jeep to provide more prisoners to work on the labour gang. All work had to be completed before our anticipated departure for Japan, rumoured to be some time in the following month. The Jeep — knowing full well that we did not have enough 'fit' men — ordered Greenpants to attend my sick parade to ensure the required number was sent to work.

'All sick on parade,' shouted the orderly sergeant. 'At the double.'

The men on parade were very ill with the usual gamut of diseases: malaria had again reared its ugly head and, in light of our virtually non-existent rations, malnutrition was becoming even worse. More and more men were sinking dangerously close to death.

With his bright green pants swishing with each sharp, short step, Greenpants approached his first sick parade. Captain Sumner, my commanding officer, asked if I needed his help. 'No thanks,' I whispered. 'I know how to deal with him.' Greenpants was one runt I did not yet fear.

The parade was called to attention and Captain Sumner handed over to Greenpants, who seemed edgy. I saluted him, as was required.

Standing by my side with the roll book in hand was Corporal Len Coon, the medical orderly from Kumi No. 36. I approached the first man on parade and, after examining him, turned to Len.

'Malaria: No Duty, five days,' I said.

Before Len had time to mark the patient's name on the roll, Greenpants yelled in Japanese: 'Not sick, work!'

The Korean was clearly determined to assert his authority in the same way he had seen Japanese Sergeant Shimojo do out on the Railway. He continued shouting and pointing to the man on parade. 'Work,' he repeated.

I explained to him, in my best pidgin Japanese, that the patient was recovering from a bout of malaria, and that his spleen was enlarged and tender. Turning my head away from Greenpants, I quickly winked at the men in line. I pressed on the patient's left upper abdomen and, on cue, he winced in mock pain. This man was genuinely ill with malaria, but I knew Greenpants would only believe a medical problem if he could see physical symptoms with his own eyes.

'You see?' I appealed.

He looked confused.

'You feel,' I said. 'I know *you* will be able to feel it.'

Greenpants stepped forward and jabbed at the patient, who once again squirmed. The Korean would never risk admitting he could not feel the spleen (which, of course, was not enlarged). His eyes were shifting; a decision needed to be made.

'Light duties in camp,' he shouted. I nodded in agreement — light duties would not cause the patient any serious harm. Another auction was under way.

This was a game of give and take: pacing was important, and I knew I had to be cautious not to push him too far. I gave in to Greenpants over several men who could cope with a day's work, careful to save my trump cards for the men who needed them most. As long as Greenpants felt as though he was in control, there was always the potential to bargain.

About halfway down the line we came to a fine young man whom I knew from the 2/15th Field Regiment, Maurice Barkley. Maurice was recovering from malaria and dysentery and, on top of this, had recently almost lost his life to pellagra.

Maurice was a remarkable young man; as a talented pianist he lived in a world of music and art; as a thinker he lived in a world of philosophy and idealism; and as a prisoner who suffered terribly from consecutive illnesses, he was somehow capable of living inside his own world, remote from pain, suffering and bitterness. At times I thought he could have walked on hot ashes or lain on a bed of nails with no concern. He would prefer to work rather than cause trouble, even if it literally cost him his life, which only made me more determined to see that he did not go to work.

'This man, very sick. If he works, he will die,' I said. Greenpants, though, was tiring of our pantomine. He shook his head. 'Work!' he screamed in Japanese.

I genuinely feared Maurice might die if he was sent to work, so I took an even harder line. 'When the war is over,' I said in pidgin Japanese. 'Prime Minister in Australia will ask why this man died. I will tell him it was because of you — you will be punished.'

I had resorted to this tactic on two previous occasions — once with The Storm Trooper and once with Sergeant Shimojo — and in both cases the guards had backed down, genuinely fearful of such consequences. But I had misread Greenpants. Suddenly his face turned red with rage and he exploded, attacking me with his boots first and then his knuckles, cursing me in Japanese.

While bashings were commonplace, this was the worst I had ever received. With each blow about the head I became increasingly dazed. I could hear Australian voices calling: 'Stay upright, Doc. Don't let the bastard knock you down or he'll get his boot into you.' More guards raced down, their fixed bayonets cutting the air. Greenpants was out of control: he kept attacking — boot, fist, boot, fist, boot, fist — in quick succession. I have no concept of how long the beating lasted, but when he finally tired he disappeared into the guardhouse, leaving me, his defeated sparring partner, bleeding in the ring.

I pushed my glasses back onto the bridge of my nose, somehow they had remained intact. Sumner quickly dismissed the sick parade and rushed to my side. I refused help from him and the other men who tried to comfort me. The heat of humiliation was rushing through me. I was furious with myself: I had overplayed my part in the game. I had become too confident and paid a painful and very public price. I wanted nothing more than to disappear.

What Maurice said as I left was blurred by the buzzing in my ears, but whatever it was it could not have been so eloquent as the look of gratitude in his eyes. While pain never seemed to reach the level of his consciousness, his profound understanding and sympathy clearly recognised suffering in others.

The water lapping onto the little beach not 50 metres away from our parade ground was inviting. It was out of camp bounds but at that point I figured I had very little left to lose. I stumbled down to the sand and dropped into the water; the salt stung my bleeding gums. I clenched my jaw and felt fragments of tooth against my tongue. Several of my teeth, including my front teeth, were broken along the edges. Cold anger surged inside me: Greenpants was a savage.

I finished bathing and then sat on some rocks at the end of the beach to dry out. Left alone with my thoughts, I contemplated my own undoing. I had enjoyed making Greenpants squirm, so much so that I had failed to retreat before he reached breaking point. I thought I knew the rules of my own game, but I had forgotten one significant factor: the reaction of a guard was never controllable. My musings were suddenly disturbed by the urgent voice of another Korean guard.

'You. Guardhouse,' he said. 'Now.'

Solitude within captivity never lasted long. I turned to face the guardhouse. It looked directly towards my forbidden bathing spot. There was no doubt in my mind The Jeep had been watching me all along. I followed the guard along the beach and back to camp.

As I climbed the steps of the guardhouse, I prepared myself

mentally for an attack from The Jeep. I hoped he would not take another swipe at my bloodied face. He was sitting in the centre of the room; on the table before him lay a bowl of fruit, a pot of tea and two small Japanese tea cups. He rose from his chair, bowed and gestured to a seat. His face did not display even a hint of aggression. What's the trick? I thought.

'Sit,' he said.

I hesitated until he pointed again. 'Sit.'

He offered me a cup of tea, an ugly smile plastered across his face. I had long before learned that it was much better to play along when dealing with guards, so I accepted with a smile, grateful for the many hours I had spent playing poker while at university. The hot tea hurt my bleeding mouth but I still had to resist the temptation to gulp it down; I was awfully thirsty and had not tasted tea for a long time. It was clearly a treat; his own version of some act of courtesy.

Still smiling at me, he pointed to the bowl on the table. 'For you,' he said.

The thought of acidic pomelos and pineapples made me shudder. Despite my hunger (I had not seen a piece of fruit since we left Saigon), I could not possibly eat a thing: my mouth was throbbing. I shook my head. 'No, thank you.'

'Like Colonel Williams, you very foolish — but very brave,' he said, and then bowed his head slightly. He was obviously imitating Naito. In my mind, there was no comparison between Colonel Williams' bravery and my own zealous self-confidence. The Jeep was just another Korean trying desperately hard to be Japanese.

'Take fruit,' he said, before dismissing me.

I finished my tea and carried the fruit out of the guardhouse, still half expecting to be swiped from behind.

I took the fruit to Len Coon at the RAP and asked him to share it among the sick. I felt sure that The Jeep knew I would do this and, in some odd way, he wanted to square off with the sick men whom he knew really were too ill to work. The tea ceremony was possibly a display of rare and brief remorse — perhaps he could sleep better at night knowing he had not personally issued my punishment, only the reward.

LATER THAT SAME DAY, Arthur Sumner and I discussed the problem of how many or how few workers we could get away with in future. We were immersed in the roll book when the orderly sergeant came bursting into the officers' area.

'Captain Richards, sir,' he said, out of breath. 'Corporal Coon needs you straight away. Two sick men have just been brought in.' The orderly sergeant's eyes were enormous, his voice animated.

'What's the trouble?' I asked, expecting dysentery or one of the other usual suspects.

'One is unconscious and the other is vomiting violently.'

I dropped the roll book and ran towards the RAP, the orderly sergeant by my side.

Inside the RAP, the unconscious patient, Corporal Gorlick, was pale and limp. He stopped breathing and started to turn blue. Despite attempts to revive him, he died within minutes. The other patient was also pale, sweating and suffering griping abdominal pains. He had already related to Corporal Coon that he and Gorlick had found some dead shellfish lying on the beach. Starving, Gorlick had tasted and swallowed the shellfish, but he had spat his out. We forced him to drink a pint of seawater to act as an emetic. His vomiting became violent, gradually ridding his body of the poisoned food.

Gorlick was the first of our men we had lost since leaving Tamarkan. On the Railway, deaths had become so common they hardly caused a ripple. In some of the cholera camps, it had not been unusual to see ten or more men being either buried or cremated on great funeral pyres every day. But now, having been away from the Railway for some months, Gorlick's death came as quite a shock and we were determined to perform his last rites in a manner more dignified than that to which we had become accustomed.

The burial ground we selected for Gorlick overlooked the calm and peaceful sea to the south. Perhaps our own subconscious preoccupation with water, which always represented the possibility, however remote, of being rescued, led us there. A grave was dug on a clearing on a small rise just beyond the parade ground. The evening light was fading when Captain Sumner, in the absence of a padre, conducted the service. He read a passage from the Bible and all men repeated with him the Lord's Prayer as the body of Corporal Gorlick, wrapped in a tattered ground sheet, was lowered into the grave. Taking their lead from Captain Sumner, all men stiffened to attention, saluted and then with bared heads, observed two minutes' silence.

THAT EVENING, THE EVENTS of the day were still spinning through my mind. Writing in my diary, it occurred to me that Gorlick might just be the ideal custodian of my papers. Only weeks away from our risky journey across the South China Sea, I was determined to see my record of events remain on dry land. Even if there was an invasion by the Allies to regain Singapore, it was unlikely Jeep Island would ever be ravaged, and there was at least a remote hope that, after the war, Gorlick's remains would be recovered and reinterred in a proper war cemetery. I resolved then and there that it was time to bury my diary summary and medical records for safekeeping.

To ensure I would never entirely lose touch with my writings, I spent the rest of the evening — until lights out — composing a brief outline of my six-and-a-half-page summary. On a single page of the thinnest piece of Japanese paper I could find, I used a sharpened pencil to enable me to write in the finest hand possible. I then rolled the summary like a cigarette and concealed it inside the tubing of my stethoscope. I thought back to my intern days at St Vincent's, when I had proudly worn my stethoscope as a status symbol to impress my patients. It certainly had a very different kind of importance now.

Two days later, I carried out the final tasks before burying my treasure. I removed the pages of my diary summary from inside a book I kept on my table and pulled from my pocket an envelope given to me the previous day by Les Stupart (who was privy to my plan, along with Len Coon and Captain Sumner). It was a Red Cross envelope addressed to Les by his parents, but on the other side he had carefully written a covering note to be buried with my records:

> This copy of Medical Records was buried by Captain C.R.B Richards on 11th August 1944 under the cross erected over the grave of Corporal Gorlick S.R. . . .

Les had listed the names, rank and unit of each of the officers located in camp, detailing that they were in command of 650 Australian, British, Dutch, American and Greek men. (To this day I have no idea about his reference to Greeks in the camp.) I placed the envelope on top of my summary, folded the pages in half and then carefully rolled them, together with the table of sickness rates and rations, into a cylinder so I could poke them through the neck of a glass bottle I had found in the guards' rubbish dump.

I packed the remainder of the bottle with paper and forced a tightly rolled wad of paper into the neck, about half an inch clear of the opening, then sealed it with molten candle grease. I hoped the seal would keep the bottle watertight for as long as necessary.

My next task was to draw a sketch map of the area so the exact site of Gorlick's grave could be plotted. If only my father could have seen me drawing such a crude but important map in my best freehand. I used an outcrop of rocks at the eastern end of the beach as a reference point and moved due west until Gorlick's grave was located due north. I marked the relative positions of the RAP, just above the outcrop, the guardhouse at the other end of the beach and the parade ground in between. I rolled up the map and slid it inside the tubing of my stethoscope, on the opposite side to my one-page summary.

Corporal Coon came rushing into the RAP later that morning to let me know that the hole for a wooden cross to mark Gorlick's grave had been dug. The Jeep had approved the building of the wooden cross and was now insisting on overseeing its erection later that day. I needed to bury my records before then.

While the midday meal was being served, I quietly slipped out behind the RAP hut with my bottle in my pocket. Darting through the undergrowth, keeping my head down, I made my way to the grave site. Just as Coon had reported, a perfectly neat hole had been dug at the head of Gorlick's grave.

I looked around and then crouched down. Using my hands, I dug the hole a little deeper in the sandy soil to accommodate my bottle. I felt surprisingly calm; perhaps comforted by the thought that at last my records would be safe. I plonked a few loose stones into the hole to keep the candle wax clear of the soil and then placed the bottle in the earth, upside down. Conscious of being away from camp for too long, I quickly packed soil around and on top of the bottle, tamping it flat with my fists. I vowed never to start another notebook; I'd had enough of diaries by then.

That night, the moment my head hit bamboo I fell into a deep sleep of utter exhaustion — and relief: carrying around my summary had been rather like holding on to a plug of dynamite with the fuse half lit. I slept peacefully, hopeful that one day both Gorlick and my records would be recovered.

CHAPTER FIFTEEN

ALL AT SEA
Voyage from Singapore
September 1944

Squinting in the sunlight, we watched natives loading rubber and other cargo onto ships. It was 5 September and we were waiting at Singapore docks to embark on our journey to Japan. The madness of having to sit beneath the tropical sun, the temperature rocketing, not even a shadow in which we could hide, is not easy to convey. Our throats were scratchy with thirst and yet there in front of us was the ocean: a covering of the coolest blue. Mentally we counted down the hours until we might enjoy the relative comfort of evening and the chance to let our skin breathe. Such empty hours of waiting provided a pit into which niggling negative thoughts could fall, at least momentarily. I looked at my watch, my only material connection to my mates; it was almost midday. I wondered what Jim and the others were up to. At times along the Railway, run off my feet, I had wished for solitude and the opportunity to be at peace with my own thoughts, surrounded by open space and free of responsibilities. But solitude is very different from loneliness, and since leaving Tamarkan I had been feeling far lonelier than I had anticipated.

Before us were two rusty cargo-passenger ships: the *Kachidoki Maru* and the *Rakuyo Maru*. Neither displayed the Red Cross or any other sign that prisoners of war would soon be onboard, only a flag, the Japanese Rising Sun — a distinct red ball in the middle of a white field, a bullseye for every Allied submarine. A row of lifeboats dangled from the decks. Both ships were similar in size and appeared equally appalling in condition.

In the afternoon, finally lined up in our *kumi* formations, we were counted off numerous times before being divided into two groups: 1000 British troops were allocated to the *Kachidoki Maru*; the remaining 600 British troops and 716 Australians (from Kumi Nos 35 to 39) to board the *Rakuyo Maru*. Our group was also joined by three senior officers: Group Captain Moore of the RAF, Colonel Harry Melton of the US Air Force and Brigadier Varley of the AIF, who were on their way to a senior officers' camp.

Ringing throughout the docks were the voices of guards: '*Hiaku, hiaku* [hurry hurry],' I heard them shout, '*bukaroo* [fool]'. *Kumi* by *kumi*, men ravaged with disease dragged themselves along the gangway of the *Rakuyo Maru*, assisted by guards pricking at their bony legs with bayonets.

Onboard, the ship's captain ordered all POWs into the holds, one of his mean fingers pointing downwards. He wore navy trousers and a matching button-up jacket; his uniform hung without discipline or pride, as if he had slept in it. He was unshaven, unkempt and clearly uninterested in our wellbeing. Immediate protests by the men were short-lived under the glint of bayonets. With the hatches not yet battened, I could peer into one of the holds: below was a dank and depressing furnace. A ladder dropped down into a small open area — a crude hallway — which led into split level 'accommodation', renovated to contain a maximum number of men. Between the two decks there was no more than a metre or so of headroom. Australians filed down the ladder of the portside hold, the Brits into the starboard hold. We were all prisoners of war but we were still very distinct forces, neither enthusiastic to interact with the other when it wasn't necessary. It seemed perfectly natural, even essential in terms of administration, for each man to remain within his own *kumi*.

Many of our men were forced to wait in the crowded hallway while those already inside the split-level decks, squatting like ducks, squeezed up to make more room. The stink of sweat was already making some retch; most were too dehydrated to vomit. With the guards congregated around the ladder, some of the men topside still waiting their turn squirrelled into hiding holes, disappearing behind lockers, below stairwells, beneath winches and anywhere else they could find. It was obvious not everyone would fit in the hold and even the blazing sun was more desirable than what they saw below.

As the guards continued to shove more and more men down the ladder, the bodies of collapsed men suffering heat exhaustion and tetany (painful muscle spasms caused by a loss of salt) began to resurface, lifted above the heads of those waiting in the hallway and passed back up to me on deck. Apart from a small stash of quinine I had no medical supplies: all I could offer was a word of encouragement and assist them in taking conservative sips from their water bottles. They were wilting, weightless in my arms; all nutrients leached from their bodies long ago.

Down below, men were being buried in bodies; it was lunacy — a callous test of the spirit of all prisoners of war — but the force of an oppressed majority can be more powerful than even armed keepers. With nothing left to lose, the flow of troops began to reverse. POWs pushed each other out of the hold and back up on deck; no longer intimidated by the prospect of a beating or a bullet. Hundreds of men emerged like front-line soldiers bursting from a trench, fury on their faces. The guards, severely outnumbered and perhaps fearing a mutiny, moved away, looking towards their grubby captain for direction.

While this commotion was taking place, Captain Sumner and Brigadier Varley, supported by John Chalmers and me, had approached Lieutenant Yamada, a fierce yet familiar face from the Railway we were almost pleased to see. Yamada followed orders but had a rare reputation for tolerance, at times even leniency, towards POWs. Sumner and Varley had pleaded with him to acknowledge the impossibility of so many men travelling below for the duration of the voyage and he had consented to inspect the hold in the company of the ship's captain, the other *kumi* commanders and medical officers.

Along with the other officers, I watched from the deck while Yamada and the captain entered the hold on the port side. The men already up on deck watched in silence, calmed by the presence of Varley and fellow officers. The captain ordered more of the remaining men out of the hold so that he and Yamada could carry out their inspection. We listened to Yamada reasoning with the captain: it was physically impossible to fit more than 1000 men into the two holds, he told him, and then added that surely they had a responsibility to deliver a certain number of live bodies at the end of their journey. Work awaited prisoners of war in Japan, Yamada reminded the captain.

The captain, no doubt anxious to get out of the stinking hold himself, relented and announced that 400 men could remain on deck, including the most seriously ill, with the other POWs permitted to be rotated between deck and hold as per a roster to be devised by the commander of each *kumi*.

Accepting the compromise as a victory, hundreds of men once again filed below deck, about 900 in total, and the guards battened the hatches. The captain refused to budge on the issue of the hatches: he maintained that if we had rain or huge seas and the hatches were open, the men would drown. The only remaining opening was on top of one of the hatches, covered by an upright structure that reminded me of a public telephone box.

Topside, I staked out a small patch at the base of the winch and established my RAP. Close by were Major Chalmers and Les Stupart. I tried to make the sick as comfortable as possible, adjusting their blankets and ensuring they had enough room to stretch out fully. We set sail at 0700 hours the following day in convoy with the *Kachidoki Maru*, two other cargo ships, two tankers and five escorts.

As we sailed out of the harbour, heading north–east towards Formosa (today known as Taiwan), I turned around for a final glimpse of Singapore Island. That phase of my life was over. Somewhere out in the South China Sea, submarines were lurking, waiting to pounce. Whatever happened next was beyond my control.

DAY AFTER DAY WHEN darkness fell, a group of us helped hundreds of men clamber from the hold to the deck. In the middle of the sea, with escape impossible, the guards were largely unconcerned with our whereabouts during the night; at times there were as many as 600 topside. During the day there was a never-ending queue for the six wooden latrines which were slung over the sides of the ship — a legitimate excuse for a break from the hold. Consisting of two planks of wood for a man to rest his feet upon and a hand rail on either side, in rough seas they posed a serious hazard. How no one ended up overboard, I can't explain.

I ran daily sick parades beneath the winch up on deck; conditions were so cramped I had to hold them progressively. In the first few days, when men below deck reported to me I detained them for as long as possible, but as the days passed, the sun became so fierce that many soon preferred to stay below, despite the darkness and the stench of urine and diarrhoea. Sailing with a slight sea breeze, the hold had become marginally cooler and it was also free from guards, who had no interest in climbing down the ladder. Throughout the day listless men surfaced from time to time to gulp a few breaths of fresh air, their eyes blinking madly, unaccustomed to the brilliance of daylight, and then disappeared again. During the evenings, the temperature dropped, and with only a single threadbare blanket to cover each man, those of us on deck were freezing. There is no pleasure in any conditions of extreme.

Our daily rations were poor: a cupful of rice topped with a watery vegetable stew if we were lucky, and a little barley; the shortage of fresh water was chronic. We had access to one sea water tap and each day the Japanese issued us with a grossly inadequate supply of fresh water. I trained a small group of volunteers to drink diluted sea water.

Long after my release from captivity, scientific types — who shall remain nameless — openly questioned that we resorted to drinking diluted sea water. In fact, I have been personally criticised for asking men to drink it. But who has the right to apply textbook advice to extraordinary circumstances, or, for that matter, to pass judgment on situations they have not lived through? When the choice on offer is an almost certain death from dehydration or learning to drink diluted sea water, I can assure the doubters that humans can adapt. We were in the middle of the South China Sea, waiting to be torpedoed, with very ill men already at risk of dying of thirst in either the stinking bowel or on the sunburned deck of a Japanese ship. Our fears of turning bonkers from excessive sodium levels were somewhat measured. The decision was pragmatic rather than radical.

Back in Changi, in our early days of captivity, we had experimented with cooking rice in sea water and had quickly learned that our palates could adjust to salt or lack of it. At sea, all of us were salt-starved. With the support of Captain Sumner and

Brigadier Varley, I suggested that a group of our men try drinking a small amount of sea water diluted with a greater amount of fresh water (a ratio of 1:2 or 3 salt water to fresh water). We gradually increased the volume of sea water, allowing our palates and stomachs to adjust until we were able to tolerate a mixture of up to 2:1 without vomiting.

On 11 September, due west of Manila, our convoy was joined by three more ships and two escorts, bringing our convoy total to seven ships, two tankers (in three rows of three) and seven escorts. Sailing in a rectangular-like formation, our ship was located in the middle of the right flank. Our convoy moved in a zigzagging pattern at all times, a standard tactic to reduce the risk of torpedo attacks. Not an hour passed without us wondering when a submarine would strike.

Following our departure from Singapore, we had constantly rehearsed in our minds our plans for abandoning ship. Officers and NCOs — especially sailors from HMAS *Perth* — instructed men, by word of mouth, to locate hatch covers and anything else wooden that could be thrown overboard and used as a raft, taking care not to drop them on men already in the sea. We were to keep our water bottles full whenever possible; wear our shirts and hats to avoid sunburn and no one was to drink sea water other than those already conditioned to it. Above all, over and over it was repeated: do not panic. Along with Major Chalmers, I was allocated responsibility for helping the sick. The other officers were in charge of disembarking the bulk of the troops from the hold. Undoubtedly at the forefront of every man's mind was his own personal plan of survival, usually in conjunction with a mate or a small group of men. My plan was simple: get the sick off first, then the men and, finally, myself. We all accepted being torpedoed as a certainty.

AT 0155 HOURS ON 12 September, after six days at sea, there was an explosion in the distance. On deck, men startled from sleep leapt up to watch one of the lead destroyer escorts in the right flank of our convoy lighting up the horizon. The sky flashed with a fantastic display of fireworks, golden splashes of yellow and dazzling orange convulsing skywards and then cascading into the sea. The remaining ships in our convoy began dropping depth charges in retaliation; the ocean rumbled around us. The racket was deafening. Within seconds, one of the oil tankers was also hit, erupting into a flaming red ball. It glowed briefly and then vanished behind masses of billowing black smoke.[1] Guards, screaming wildly, appeared on deck, firing their rifles in all directions but at nothing in particular. For once their agitation was not directed towards us. POWs started clambering out of the holds, but there wasn't a stampede: this was the moment we had been expecting. Most joined us on deck to watch the electric sky-show.

Time passes in a deceptive fashion in a battle zone. In recollecting events, I remember the order and number of explosions but not the specific amount of time that lapsed in between. Official naval records show that the next torpedo did not strike our convoy until 0524 hours, when an oil tanker directly to the left of our ship exploded. This means we spent about three and a half hours up on deck, watching the sky. I felt strangely calm during that time, fascinated by the explosions and replaying in my mind the abandon ship procedures we had been practising. Perhaps my sense of responsibility and duty blotted out dormant fear. The guards began erratic firing again just after the tanker was hit. I wondered how long it would be before our turn came.

It came immediately. One of our lads, looking out from the starboard side, screamed that he could see the white trails of torpedoes speeding towards us. 'They're coming!' he yelled, and within moments we were hit: one forward and one amidships, both striking just below the water line. It was only when I recalled the incident later that I clearly remembered, first, noticing the dull thuds of the torpedoes hitting, one after the other, several seconds apart; second, the engine of the ship ceasing to throb; and third, a towering wave sweeping over the deck. One. Two. Three. But at the time all three seemed to happen at once. I clung to the mast and watched my water bottle and haversack disappear overboard. Inside my haversack was my stethoscope: my one-page diary summary was lost at sea, but my waterproof wallet containing my pay book, photos, letters from home and other papers remained snug in my shirt pocket.

Here memories shift in between actual events and thoughts contaminated by the passage of time. I can remember clear flashes amongst patches of uncertainty, but what I can say, beyond doubt, is that there was no panic amongst our men. Did I think this would be the end for us? No — maybe I was a slow learner. It is difficult for others to understand how a rational response can be applied in situations where most would expect pandemonium. Over the years I have been asked repeatedly, 'Are you in denial? Torpedoed and yet no panic?' The askers of such questions have usually failed to understand that even though we had been hit, we did not appear to be sinking, nor were we going up in flames like the other ships before us. We were also trained and disciplined soldiers. We had time to gather our thoughts and turn our minds to the evacuation plan we had so often rehearsed. There was fear, yes, but not panic: the two can remain very separate.

The torpedo activity continued; the ship directly in front of ours had also been hit. The guards, ignoring us completely, lowered all lifeboats into the sea, except for two which seemed to be jammed. The Japanese abandoned ship within ten minutes of the torpedoes hitting, leaving behind most of their supplies and even some of their bayonets. The captain certainly wasn't going down with his ship; he was the very first to jump. I recall his blue rowboat vividly because in it were not only the captain and the ship's cabin boy but also one of our own men, an Australian gunner. It was the most un-Australian display of character I have ever witnessed; his wrongdoing made all the greater for the fact that he was prepared to leave his brother onboard while he saved his own skin. Why the captain allowed a prisoner of war in his boat, I do not know, but the arrangement didn't last long — the lad soon ended up in the sea with the rest of the men, clinging to debris. At the time, I was disgusted by his behaviour, but in my later years, looking back, it is not for me to condemn others. It is true he valued his own life above that of his brother and mates, but that is something he had to live with for the rest of his life. He survived and his brother did not.

On deck, after the wave had passed over us, as far as I could see none of our men had been washed overboard, nor had any been badly injured. Others later told me of Japanese deaths. I saw none but there must have been some: those in the engine room surely lost their lives in an instant. Major Chalmers and I helped other men on deck remove heavy covers from the holds. We pitched them overboard and then ordered sick men to jump and swim to the floating hatches. A few were so weak they needed a gentle push, but most didn't need too much encouragement: the torpedo activity around us continued and we all knew we were still a sitting target for another strike. Australians evacuated on the port side, the Brits from starboard. The drop into the sea from the deck was about six metres. Men tumbled overboard, their bodies seemingly disappearing, curving backwards and inwards towards the ship as it kept moving forward. Jack McKone, an older man of the 2/15th Field Regiment who had also been assisting me with the sick, disappeared into the Japanese quarters to replace lost water bottles and supplies. Perhaps by now our ship was beginning to sink, but we knew we were not about to be sucked down into the belly of the ocean just yet.

By daylight, most men had been evacuated and only about a dozen of us remained. We were determined to launch the two remaining lifeboats that the Japanese had left behind. We tried to move the one on the port side but the davits were rusted; we couldn't budge it. We then checked the one on the starboard side and discovered the same problem. Some more of the boys in the water swam back to the ship to help us, while others chose to depart. Further torpedo attacks in the area frightened off some of the men, who decided to take their chances and jump overboard to the safety of a raft, including fellow officers Jim Burke, Les Stupart and Campbell Smith. This left me as the only remaining officer onboard. I was prepared to take a calculated risk that it was safer to secure a lifeboat, into which many of us could fit, than take my chances stranded on a piece of floating wood.

We managed to force the davits to release the starboard lifeboat; it dropped suddenly but with shortened ropes it was left suspended well above water level. A couple of men obtained bayonets from the Japanese quarters and used them to hack at the ropes like a woodchopper with an axe. The lifeboat crashed into the water and we jumped overboard after it, taking with us a couple of five-gallon tins of water and some biscuits which had also been lifted from Japanese quarters. Upon impact some of the planks inside the boat were sprung and the boat was soon leaking.

It is peculiar the minute details you can recall later while more important moments remain blank: I do not remember the names or faces of all the men I jumped overboard with, but I can still picture the bright blue waste cloth we found inside the lifeboat — where it came from, God only knows, but we used it to pack the leaks. We took turns in bailing out water using tin buckets. Once the leaks were under control, we rowed towards some of our men who were swimming in our immediate area and collected as many passengers as we could — one of whom was a Japanese prostitute whose keepers had so nobly left behind. She sat quietly, I remember her pink lips and her face, pale and frightened. It was heartening to see the chivalry of the boys who were prepared to cling to the edges of our boat to let her remain sitting inside. We had some 60 odd survivors in and around the lifeboat; only about fifteen inside due to the leaking.

Debris surrounded us and in between were men, hanging on to anything that floated. Some had drowned — many could not swim — and others had been killed by falling wreckage from rigging. I was later told by others that a select few of the POWs had resorted to taking revenge on some of the guards, holding their heads under water until they drowned or attacking them with bayonets they had taken from the ship. I did not see any such encounters, most of us were far too busy trying to survive for revenge to even enter our minds, yet I cannot say these acts did not take place. I only remain thankful that I did not have to witness them. Every man responds differently in difficult situations. At the other end of the spectrum was Jimmy Mullens, a lifesaver from Manly. For Jimmy, being stranded in the sea was an opportunity to celebrate his own liberation. I can still picture him swimming backwards and forwards between the rafts, playful like a porpoise — cheerful to be free to splash in the ocean, the place he loved like no other.

Throughout the morning we remained in the vicinity of the *Rakuyo Maru*. It was still afloat but by now well on its way to going down, the rising sea washing over the deck. In the distance, the Japanese in lifeboats remained in their own cluster, keeping well out of reach of desperate prisoners of war who might try to clamber onboard. All around us hundreds of men were hanging onto rafts or struggling to keep swimming. We, too, had to keep our distance from our own men, using our oars to row away from their reach. We had as many passengers as we could safely hold, any more and we risked all going down.

The remaining Japanese ships in our convoy continued to drop depth charges; our lifeboat shuddered with the force of each explosion. Just before midday, one of the Japanese lifeboats rowed towards us. The guards on board were armed; we were not.

Naturally we feared they wanted to turf us from our lifeboat to claim it for themselves, but it was our water and rations they wanted, along with their little 'popsy'. The Japanese woman climbed into their lifeboat and there was nothing else we could do to help her. We were forced to hand over all the supplies they could see, but thankfully one of the water tins and a stash of biscuits had been concealed in the nick of time. We breathed a sigh of relief when they rowed away from us, content with their pillage.

LATE IN THE AFTERNOON, we were drifting about two kilometres from the *Rakuyo Maru* when it finally sank. Some thought the rubber cargo helped it stay afloat for so long (about twelve hours in total). In the questioning of fellow survivors after the war, 50 per cent of men claim it sank by the bow, the other half swear it sank by the stern, and yet we all witnessed it disappear into the sea. I cannot with absolute confidence say which way it was. My money has always been on bow first, but whose memory is actually correct is anyone's guess.

At dusk, two unharmed Japanese frigates from our original convoy appeared, easing their way amongst the debris to search for survivors. Initially we hoped we might be rescued but such hopes were fleeting. When a few prisoners of war tried to scramble up the nets of the frigate, the Japanese immediately flicked them back into the ocean, like fisherman rejecting small fish. It was clear we were not going to be picked up. The rescuers plucked their own men to safety and disappeared as quickly as they had arrived, leaving all of us in the closing darkness. Rather than disappointment I think my reaction was relief: at least they had chosen to leave us stranded rather than shooting us up, the lesser of two evils at the time. Perhaps because of their haste to get out of the area, the guards had left their abandoned lifeboats in the ocean. It seemed a minor miracle; at the very least we had expected the guards to blast the lifeboats or shoot holes in them. I doubt it had been an intended act of courtesy.

We recovered all ten of the Japanese boats, we could fit about 30 to 40 men inside each, and we replaced our leaking boat with one of the released boats. A few men decided to take their chances and remained on the leaking boat. With only a few onboard they deemed they could control the leaking and keep it afloat. During the afternoon, some of the POWs had swum back to the *Rakuyo Maru* and were successful in their attempts to free the remaining lifeboat. Including this boat, the leaking boat and the ten abandoned Japanese boats we had a total of twelve, but there were still not enough to save all men and we had to leave behind the men on rafts whom we knew were scattered somewhere in the distance. At the time it was a question of survival. A fundamental rule of first aid is not to expose yourself or others to further danger; we had to do what was best for the group we were with. It is a situation in which no man would ever wish to be placed: one in which you have to think with your head rather than heart in order to save the maximum number of lives.

By this time, I was seasick — not just a little nausea, but fair dinkum seasick, the kind where you actually want to die. To have lived through so many horrors on the Railway only to wish my life away to such an ailment was pitiful. Hour after hour we had been bobbing up and down, drifting. I will forever regret that I was too ill to say goodbye to my friends, Corporal Len Coon, the medical orderly of Kumi No. 36 who had been such a help to me on Jeep Island, and Lieutenant Campbell Smith, commander of Kumi No. 39 whom I also knew from Anderson Force. When their boat drifted within speaking distance of ours, they had called out to speak to me. I was so ill I could barely raise an eyebrow, let alone sit up to wish them luck. I heard another voice calling from their boat, telling us they intended to sail east to the Philippines. Someone from our boat told them we had decided to sail west to

China. They seemed happy to go their own way, equipped with sails, drinking water, biscuits and cigarettes. No man from that boat was ever seen again.

We remained within calling distance of two other boats which had also decided on China as their intended destination. During the night, we tied our boats together with rope, stem to stern. With a squally wind blowing up from the east we gave up on the idea of rowing as it would only waste energy and the wind would carry us overnight. Two rowers per boat were detailed in two-hour shifts to keep the boats from banging into one another. I started to feel better once our boat stopped wallowing and started moving forward. A compass was found on one of the lifeboats but the lighting apparatus was faulty, rendering it largely useless during the night. Instead, we adopted a far more practical method: steering by the stars throughout a cloudless night. My prewar experience with the Survey Regiment proved valuable, as I recognised some of the constellations but have now forgotten their names.

By about 3.00 a.m., I could barely keep my eyes open. I explained to one of the lads how to follow the appropriate star, gave him my watch, Jim's gift, to wear on his thin wrist and asked him to wake me in an hour. While I slept the lad hung his arm over the side. The catch slipped and the watch plonked into the ocean. He wakened me in a fretful state to inform me of the loss. He was terribly upset, stuttering his explanation.

I didn't need to make him feel any worse than he already did. 'Never mind,' I said. 'Just don't lose an oar.' I lay back and closed my eyes, unspeakably saddened.

AT SUNRISE THE FOLLOWING day, we redistributed ourselves among the three boats so that mates could be with mates and then decided to cut our boats adrift. With the sea becoming more choppy the risk of bumping into each other and damaging a boat was too great and with our boats scattered we were convinced we stood a better chance of being noticed by any submarine that surfaced. I found myself on a boat with five other AIF men, Jack McKone (my helper during the evacuation of the sick), Kitch Loughnan, Lindsay Savage, Ian MacDiarmid, and Manly lifesaver Jimmy Mullens. Also onboard were some lads from HMAS *Perth* as well as British RN men. We appointed a quartermaster and he had under his direct control the water, biscuits, cigarettes and tobacco. There was enormous value in having *Perth* survivors with us who were well trained in what could go wrong at sea (they had already survived one shipwreck). As a precaution, they requested that the quartermaster also collect all knives (our eating irons and pen knives) in the boat in case any one 'ran amok'. Any man who loses his mind at sea is capable of the unimaginable.

Later in the morning, on the northern horizon, we saw a convoy of the other eight lifeboats (including the leaking boat) tied one behind the other. Brigadier Varley, John Chalmers and Arthur Sumner were somewhere amongst them. One of their boats sailed in our direction and eventually joined us, bringing our group total to four. We estimated that our trip to the China coast would probably take ten to twelve days, so we calculated a daily ration of biscuits and cigarettes per man. We allowed a ration of a quarter of a pint of water morning and night and, in addition, those of us who had learned to drink salt water also did so. Our boat was equipped with a piece of canvas which we used as both a sail and to collect water every time there was a shower of rain. It was our intention to live up to our anticipated rainwater income and to save the one five-gallon cask for an emergency.

Thinking back it now seems somewhat bewildering that in the midst of being stranded at sea we spoke of preparing for an emergency, as if our circumstances at that time were not already worthy of being deemed as such! But that was the way it was, preparing for the next big thing enabled us to keep focusing on a future existence.

Sailing in a westerly direction all day, by the afternoon I began to experience a sense of freedom for the first time in two and a half years. Moving before a lovely breeze, the sea calm, all of us breathing clean air and enjoying a portion of dry biscuit, we remained positively convinced that we were advancing towards China. We had not lost hope, but by this point we were not denying reality either. I think we were all silently placing a two-bob each-way bet on our survival. We soon found ourselves slipping into a rare mood of reminiscence, passing hour after hour discussing the Malayan campaign and the tragedy it became. We remembered the night capitulation was announced; the march to Changi; our much-loved concert parties and the countless activities in which we engaged our minds to retain sanity. We remembered the formation of 'A' Force, rumours of being sent home, the trip from the aerodrome at Tavoy to the jungles of Burma. The diseases, the suffering and the madness.

Our darker thoughts were tempered with recollections of the sheer beauty of Burma: her rosy red dawns, shadowy hills of all shades of green, gigantic teak trees and the loveliness of a freshly picked orchid. We relived the humorous with the tragic, times of famine and others of relative plenty. But above all else, we remembered our mates who were no longer with us: those lost at sea, or who died in the Railway death camps and those killed in action. The past flickered through our minds, reeling from one moment to the next. Never before had I indulged in so much nostalgia and it was a rare pleasure to share our experiences without despair or bitterness.

Perhaps at that moment, free of our captors and with the opportunity to linger in the solace of so many memories, we were luckier than those we had left behind in the working parties on dry land.

CHAPTER SIXTEEN

RESCUED
South China Sea to Tokyo
September 1944

Early on the morning of our third day at sea, the sun already high in the sky, we were startled by the sound of uninterrupted gunfire. It seemed to be coming from somewhere to the north of our group of four boats. Having lost sight of the seven other lifeboats (the Varley group), our immediate fear was that these men had just been gunned down by a Japanese ship. Up until that moment, our spirits had remained high, still revelling in our own sense of freedom and steadfast in the belief that we were on course to reach China. But now, all of a sudden, we were entering dark times again: more of our mates were presumed dead — and we would probably be next.

I don't remember how we spent the hour or so that passed in between when we heard the gunfire and then watched as a Japanese frigate, followed by two corvettes, appeared over the horizon, but I do recall, once again, that there was no panic amongst us. A calm fatalism came into play. We simply accepted that our time had come. We hoped that our end would be quick and merciful, but we made a pact that if any man was severely wounded and unable to take care of himself, then any other survivors were to put him out of his misery. None of us wanted to be a burden on our mates. Then we simply said our goodbyes, shook hands and waited. Whatever the outcome, we were quietly comforted by the knowledge that we were all in this together.

It might seem far-fetched that we could be so composed in the face of death, but we were all men of an era vastly different from the emotionally effusive world of today. Our control reflected the fact that we still considered ourselves — first and foremost, and during every day of captivity — as disciplined soldiers. Our reaction was highly organised and instinctively military. Looking back now, the sense of quiet courage amongst the men onboard these boats was not something we were necessarily taught or had simply learned. It was a combination of mentally overcoming petrifying fear (after all, every one experiences fear) and allowing discipline, training, experience and even instinct to take over. In the military, it seemed natural for us to think this way.

As the frigate approached the first boat in our little cluster, its guns clearly manned and pointing towards it, those of us in the other three boats lowered our heads and waited for the loud drum of gunfire. The expectation was awful. All I could hear was the sound of my own heart thudding. I noticed the burned lips of some of the men around me moving in silent prayer.

Minutes passed and there was no gunfire. We slowly lifted our gaze to see our own lads scrambling up the netting on the side of the frigate. They looked like stick insects, their bony limbs moving quickly against the rope. My immediate reaction was suspicion; it had to be a trap. Perhaps after being interrogated our boys would be shoved overboard or shot. The idea that this might be a genuine rescue seemed impossible. The frigate quickly picked up speed and moved towards the next boat.

Our boatload was the last to clamber onboard, and to my great joy my misgivings about the rescue were proved wrong. We found the rest of our men from the other three boats huddled in the bow of the ship: 80 Australians and 56 Brits. Guards were posted around us. They made it clear we were to sit quietly or we would be turned over to the sailors who wore machine-guns slung across their chests. Sitting on the deck, beneath the blazing sun, all men suffering severe sunburn, dysentery and dehydration, their lips cracked and bleeding, blisters on their skin, we were elated. The intense excitement in finding friends safely onboard outweighed every discomfort or any immediate concern about what might come next.

Only recently I have read in a fellow survivor's account that it was Lieutenant Yamada who had prevailed upon the captain of this frigate to return to the area near the site of the torpedo attack to pick up POW survivors. Russell Savage (of the 2/10th Field Regiment) records in *A Guest of the Emperor* that Yamada did this not for humanitarian reasons but in order to carry out his own orders to deliver a work gang to Japan; that the Japanese lieutenant feared grave consequences of arriving in his homeland empty-handed.[1] This is a possibility but not a fact I have ever been able to verify. I believe our rescue could even have been an act of compassion on Yamada's part. We could have been left at sea or shot in our lifeboats, but someone made the decision to come back for us, and I will always wonder who it was.

As the only Australian officer amongst my men, I requested to see the Japanese commander of the ship. He was a fresh-faced young man and he did not seem hostile. In pidgin Japanese I asked him what had happened to Varley's group of seven boats. He seemed to understand and pointed to the other corvettes in his convoy. At the time I believed he was indicating that the others had been rescued before us by the corvettes and we were greatly relieved. During the day, and until the early hours of the following morning, we sailed generally in a western direction, zigzagging. The guards provided us with army-type dry biscuits and approximately half a litre of fresh water each.

While we rested against one another on the decks, little did we know that US submarines were about to surface near the site of the sinking of the *Rakuyo Maru,* where we had left behind our mates stranded on rafts. I can only imagine what these men must have felt, not just to be rescued, but rescued by Allied forces. The term of their captivity had finally come to an end. Between the afternoon of the fourth day and the evening of the sixth, all of the remaining raft survivors were rescued by the American submarines. Not all of the men from the rafts made it; many had died during the days they were stranded, mostly from drowning, malaria or madness. Reportedly a total of 92 Australian former POWs from the *Rakuyo Maru* eventually made it home to relay the horrible truth about our experiences on the Railway and the torpedo attacks.[2]

I later learned that following the arrival of these rescued men in Australia, my parents had been invited to a memorial service for me at the Cenotaph in Martin Place, Sydney. They declined to attend. They had been told three different versions of how I had died. Newspapers reported that the Japanese had left POW survivors to drown, and certainly no one in Australia was aware that any Japanese ships had also returned to the area to pick up POW survivors. My mother steadfastly chose to disbelieve all accounts and, as if to enforce her belief that I was still alive, on the day of the service she fetched my best evening clothes from my wardrobe — a dinner jacket and tails — and hung them out in the sun to air, ready for my return. She refused to accept that I wasn't coming home. Of course, I was thankfully ignorant of all of this until after the war. The thought of loved ones waiting for me kept me going. If I had known at the time that anyone at home presumed me dead, it would have been soul destroying.

MID-MORNING THE FOLLOWING DAY, 15 September, we came in sight of land. At first we thought it was China but, in fact, it was the large Chinese island of Hainan To (at the time occupied by the Japanese). Our frigate steamed into the harbour and we were ordered to disembark onto an oil tanker. The other two corvettes that had been some distance behind us came closer and we searched in vain for any sign of Varley and his men. I again asked the Japanese commander what had happened to Varley's group of lifeboats; he again pointed to the other corvettes. Whether he knew that the other boats had been shot up, or whether he did not understand me, or perhaps this was his own way of being polite, I will never know. Varley's group of boats was never seen again nor, to my knowledge, has any evidence ever surfaced to suggest the absolute truth of their fate. Those of us who heard the gunfire shortly before we were rescued have only ever believed that their end was swift.

Onboard the oil tanker we were shocked to discover 520 British troops who had been on the *Kachidoki Maru*.[3] The sight and smell of burned flesh is not something anyone can try to imagine; it's beyond comprehension. We learned that they had been torpedoed late in the evening on the same day we had been struck. (By the time they were attacked our lifeboats had drifted well beyond sight or hearing distance.) Many of the 1000 Brits on board went down with the ship, which sank within twenty minutes of the strike. The men who made it overboard remained in the water for at least 24 hours — swimming or floating in a heavy oil slick — before being picked up by a flotilla of small boats from nearby Hainan To, which carried them back to a Japanese oil tanker in the harbour. Again I wondered who ordered the rescue which, initially, seemed to be more compassionate than pragmatic. Now before us they were all coated in oil, which had penetrated their eyes and ears causing excruciating pain and blindness. Most suffered severely from oil burns and sunburn in addition to some with broken limbs.

Moaning in agony, men lay beneath the shade of the ship's bridge. Those who couldn't fit were forced to lie in direct sunlight on the exposed decks. We moved among these men to assess their condition and render what limited first aid was possible. The Japanese refused to provide medical supplies or any other form of assistance except for a bucket and a length of rope. In the absence of fresh water we had to use sea water to try to wipe oil from their eyes, skin and matted hair. Their skin looked as if it had melted, blisters erupting in patches. There was anguish on the face of each of these men. The decks on the tanker were steel and as hot as hell. Little could be done until after sunset; their burned eyes and skin could barely tolerate our touch beneath the sun. With their disfigured faces and scorched bodies these men were the living dead.

The stench of their burned skin was ghastly. I reached my physical limit of tolerance at about ten- to fifteen-minute intervals, when I would have to move away to vomit and breathe in some fresh air for a minute or two before being able to return to the men. The situation was impossible: we had no supplies to cope with their injuries and the Japanese refused my repeated requests to move the men onto land into some form of hospital accommodation.

The following day, still docked in the harbour at Hainan To, we were ordered to move yet again: this time onto a converted whaling mother ship, the *Kibitsu Maru*. It was torture for the unfortunate wretches who were unable to open their eyes, they had to be led by our boys, who acted as surrogate guide dogs. By late afternoon all men had been transferred and we left Hainan To Harbour, bound for Japan. It had now been four days since we were sunk. Only 136 of us from the *Rakuyo Maru* and approximately 520 from the *Kachidoki Maru* had been saved by the Japanese: a total of approximately 656 POWs out of more than 2300.[4]

The whaling mother ship consisted of one great open deck just above water level, with a trap door in the stern and numerous rails across the deck, obviously where the whales used to be hauled aboard and moved on trucks. This ship had presumably been converted during wartime for the use of landing craft. Generally the ship was in good order, the crew, as much as we saw of them, appeared to move about efficiently and purposefully. The skipper was brisk in his movements and looked almost naval in his demeanour (it was rumoured he had served in the Japanese Navy during the First World War). All the Japanese wore life jackets. Also onboard were a large number of Japanese survivors from the torpedoed ships. I recall a brief and unspoken feeling of understanding between us and this group of Japanese men. For once we had something in common: we were all survivors. They remained topside while we piled down into the bow section of the hold of the ship. Human freight on yet another journey.

The hold extended the full length of the ship and each man was allocated a space of about 80 centimetres wide and three metres long, enough room to lie down and stretch out on a grass mat. Down below it was dark, the faces of men dully illuminated by a few ceiling lights; daylight filtered through the hatch only. While conditions were awful, the burned men were relieved to at least be out of the sun. We segregated the very ill men into a separate group to make it easier to attend to them. Still denied medical supplies we maintained treatment of wiping them with sea water and offering kindly words of encouragement.

There was no provision for ablution in the hold and up on deck there were only four wooden latrines slung over the side of the ship to cater for over 650 prisoners onboard, nearly all of whom were suffering from diarrhoea or dysentery. Only those using the latrines were allowed on deck. Sentries manned the top of the gangway, vigilant in preventing any of us from going topside before another man returned from the latrine. Many were not well enough to climb the ladder out of the hold and were forced to use a bucket. We would never become accustomed to living with the stench of human waste.

Meal times were like feeding displays at a zoo. Food was lowered into the hold in a bucket on the end of a rope. We were fed mainly rice with a spoonful of vegetable stew and a little meat and barley. Nearly all men had lost their haversacks overboard so without our eating irons we had to take turns using our fingers to scoop a little food from the bucket and sip water from another communal bucket. It was yet another example of the capacity of our keepers to endlessly deny us the most basic of human dignities.

Empty 44-gallon drums lined the walls of the hold. Loosely tied with chains or some type of wire rope, they rattled and clanged unbearably loudly as the ship moved. The rest and sleep we longed for was impossible. There were numerous alarms, the wailing of air-raid sirens, and what appeared to be gun drills by the Japanese. With every sign of activity above us our hearts began to beat just a little faster in anticipation of another torpedo attack. Our ship moved in company with three other transports, and we were escorted by three small frigates. After two or three days we found ourselves in the midst of a typhoon; the swell of the sea was incredible. Each time the ship lurched the 44-gallon drums bashed against the sides of the ship, the echo so great that every crash sounded like an explosion. The naval men amongst us listened carefully to the rhythm of the ship's engines. I remember several times when the throbbing of the engines appeared to falter, the naval men calling out 'She's dropped revs', making us sure we had been hit.

Two of the transport ships were reportedly badly damaged during the typhoon and one of the frigates remained with these damaged ships, reducing our convoy to a total of four. After four days at sea, we pulled in to Keeloon, Formosa, where we remained docked for five days before departing for Japan. We all held grave doubts that we would make it to the 'land of milk and honey' in one piece. Sirens continued to wail and we remained constantly on edge. With only one ladder to exit the hold we knew our chances of surviving an attack this time around would be close to non-existent.

A day or two later, when we estimated we were only a further day or so away from reaching Japan, we found ourselves in the midst of another torpedo attack. It was the middle of the night and those of us down below saw an amazing flash of light beaming through the hatch as one of the frigates went up in flames. We were told by men who were up on deck at the time that it sank within minutes. Another thunderous explosion followed when the other transport was hit. That left two of us: one frigate and our whaling mother ship. We proceeded in a zigzag fashion on our way to Japan, the tension increasing as we came closer to land. By this stage our nerves were well beyond frayed. We expected death every moment. The constant anticipation of a torpedo attack was a far more powerful tormenter than our keepers could ever hope to be.

AT LAST, ON 28 September, about mid-afternoon, the Japanese saw land. We could hear their excited voices up on deck, joyous to be so close to their homeland. Some were so jubilant they climbed down into the hold and handed their life jackets to us. The sentries at the top of the gangway were now happy to share a joke and let a number of us up on deck, me included. There before us was the spectacle of a beautiful tree-lined shore. The sight of the pine trees reminded me of Manly beach, and at that very moment I remember experiencing a fleeting sense that I, too, was heading home.

My thoughts of home were interrupted abruptly when suddenly, only a couple of kilometres from land, the ship heeled, turning at an acute angle from the shore. Those of us up on deck were startled to see the telltale white wake of two torpedoes speeding towards our ship. Every man on deck sobered in an instant. I was not confident that our sluggish ship could heel hard enough to avoid the torpedoes. There was nothing we could do but stand there and watch, holding our breaths.[5]

The ship turned sufficiently and the two torpedoes passed harmlessly in front of us, literally only metres away. So many near misses left us mentally shattered and utterly exhausted. As we proceeded up the coast we all wondered whether there were any more submarines lying in wait on the beach. Many of the Japanese — still in a state of panic — demanded that we hand back their life jackets. It is perplexing to me that there is no record of this near miss. Official naval records do not confirm that this event took place, but I saw it with my own eyes.

We finally moved into the Japanese harbour of Moji at dusk, bringing an end to our twelve-day journey. Only eight men had died during the trip and all deaths were from previous injuries: exposure, dysentery, burns and exhaustion.[6] As each man died we had wrapped his frail body in a Japanese straw mat, carried him up on the deck and, with permission from the sentries, dropped our comrade into the ocean with due reverence and a prayer. It is remarkable that so few of these desperately ill and injured men died during such a horrendous journey. I think most of the oil-burned Brits, numbed with pain, were almost beyond caring if they lived or died. Perhaps some had gone past the stage of actively wanting to die or maybe the fact that they had been rescued gave some an even greater determination to live. Whatever the reasons, the survival rate was nothing short of miraculous.

My recollection of stepping onto dry land again is a blur only. Relief certainly, which is perhaps an oversimplification of an emotion I cannot recall. We had no idea what we were in for next and at that particular moment we didn't care; as long as we were on dry land again we at least stood a chance of making it. Some people have asked me if it was difficult to physically stand on land again after so long at sea. I think many of the very ill men were so weak it was difficult for them to stand at all, but the opportunity to escape further torpedo attacks was incentive enough for all of us to somehow stumble ashore.

Dressed only in the stinking remnants of clothing in which we had jumped overboard, we were freezing. Some, including me, wore a shirt and shorts while others wore only a tattered G-string. Quite a number of Australians had managed to retain their slouch hats. The Japanese split our group of 650 into four parties: one of 300 British under Captain Wilkie (of Straits Settlement Volunteer Force) was to go to Yokahama; one of 50 Australians was to be sent separately to Yokahama; a group of ten who were too sick to travel were to remain in Moji for later admission to hospital and the remaining 290 troops, me included, were to be under the command of Captain Peirce (Royal Artillery), bound for Sakata — known as 22D camp. I immediately complained vigorously to the Japanese that the group of 80 Australians should not be separated but my protests were shrugged off. To be detached from fellow Australian mates and find ourselves under British command was galling.

Our group was ordered to march to some horse stables nearby. Inside, the wooden walls provided evidence that other POWs had been there ahead of us. There were several names and army numbers carved into the woodwork, including the units from which they came. The next day we were each issued with one blanket and then herded onto a train being taken, we understood, to Tokyo. This was the day on which one of the most pitiless and degrading experiences of my time in captivity occurred.

Barefooted and with only a blanket wrapped around our shoulders we were forced to shuffle through the streets of Tokyo surrounded by locals. Men were so weak and bone-thin they could barely stand upright; many had lost control over their bowels and their blanket and skin were stained with defecation.

Some of the locals seemed stunned by our condition, their mouths agape; others chose to jeer and laugh loudly as we passed them by, clutching onto our blankets. This was almost too much for any man to endure, but for those of us who still had the strength, the taunting encouraged us to hold our heads up and look straight ahead in defiance, determined not to reveal our utter humiliation — which was bordering on despair. Listening to the sound of fellow humans laughing at our suffering remains one of the lowest moments of my life.

CHAPTER SEVENTEEN

SAKATA[1]
October 1944–June 1945

From Tokyo we travelled in passenger carriages to Sakata, a harbour town on the far north-west coast of Honshu, directly opposite Siberia. My brain remained so numb from the undignified march in Tokyo that I barely remember anything of this journey.

Upon arrival in Sakata our group stood in line, awaiting orders. Our shrunken bodies resembled those of fragile old men; ribs jutting out, covered only in thinly stretched skin. We had by now been issued with three blankets, a worsted suit, an overcoat (British captured stock), a pair of thin cotton socks, a second-hand pair of long underpants, a second-hand shirt and a pair of well-worn boots. The boots were much too small for at least half the men. This was to be our modest winter wardrobe in outside temperatures that would soon dive as low as minus 30 to 40 degrees Celsius.

We were allocated yet another POW number: I was given No. 6, not that it much mattered; it was just another number. Two Japanese civilian doctors attended the medical examinations conducted by Jim Roulston (a Brit and my fellow medical officer) and me. I cannot recall their names — one was a surgeon, the other a physician — but I clearly remember that they treated us all with respect; it was a pleasant surprise. They recorded our height, chest circumference, weight, foot length (which we hoped might mean we would receive new shoes) and age. More than half our group were affected by skin infections related to sun and oil burns; some had corneal ulcers and nearly all suffered from one or more of malaria, diarrhoea and oedema from beriberi and protein deficiency. The average weight of our men was calculated as 58.3 kilograms; most had lost at least ten kilograms, some as much as twenty kilograms, since commencing the sea journey to Japan.

We were accommodated in a local school while permanent billets were being built for us and here we spent three days resting before the men were forced to labour once more. Physically debilitated and mentally devastated, they were clearly unfit to work. The Imperial Japanese Army had leased, or rather 'flogged off', our group to a large stevedoring and manufacturing conglomerate, the Nippon Tsun Company. We were to be fed and supposedly cared for by this firm in return for our labour.

I was not particularly at home in the company of my fellow officers, all of whom were Brits. Our commanding officer, Captain J.E. 'Tam' Peirce, and the adjutant/quartermaster, Captain Dick Pote-Hunt, were both regular British Army officers and they brought with them all their prejudices against 'colonials', as they called all Australians. I struggled to find anything in common with them. Fortunately the other two officers, Captain Bill Barrett, the works officer, and Captain Jim Roulston were both members of the Territorial Army, similar to Australia's Militia, and they were far more likeable and egalitarian companions.

I continued in my role as medical officer, sharing the workload with Jim Roulston, and at long last we were able to practise medicine with medicine. The IJA issued us with a case of essential medical supplies and equipment — scalpels, scissors, probes, forceps and various medicines. After having had virtually no medical supplies for two and a half years this was paradise — and as an added bonus they also gave us a cupboard in which to store everything! We were allocated a 'hospital' area which could comfortably accommodate ten patients, although we usually had between twelve and sixteen men in confinement at any one time. With no heating we suspended blankets from ill-fitting windows and doors to try to prevent draughts.

Our camp was under the command of Lieutenant Watanabe and about twelve other guards from a local IJA unit. None of these men had previous experience in dealing with prisoners of war and they were not brutal towards us. Civilian employees of Nippon Tsun, in control of the men during work hours, were not, however, averse to issuing physical punishment. (Although, in comparison to what we had experienced on the Railway, beatings were occasional rather than daily — a small mercy for which we were grateful.)

Hours of work for the men were mostly from 0630 to 1700 hours with a break of one and a half hours for lunch and a half hour break morning and evening. The labour consisted of three types: filling and moving trucks in and around a chemical factory; unloading coal from barges and loading it into railway wagons; and dismantling rafts of timber in the water and loading timber on the railway wagons. Heavy work for starved and far from supple muscles. The men were paid at a rate of 10 cents a day with an extra 5 cents for NCOs and an extra 15 cents for WOs but with no canteen facilities there were few opportunities for spending. I conducted daily sick parades, tending to the 29 Australians and helping Jim care for the 260 Brits. Jim and I were responsible for supplying the required number of daily workers to Nippon Tsun. There was constant pressure to deliver enough men, but nowhere near what it had been like on the Railway — I received no bashings when negotiating on behalf of the sick.

But while the violence had subsided, our food situation was dire: we were surviving on what were frighteningly scant rations for men already in such poor health. Most meals consisted of approximately a half litre of a runny mixture of rice and vegetables. Often the only 'vegetable' present was seaweed and some other form of obnoxious vegetable which we could not identify. Captain Peirce and I wrote a formal letter to Lieutenant Watanabe soon after our arrival. We explained that even when the men were undertaking heavy work in Burma and Thailand they had been accustomed to receiving a greater ration of rice and stew than what they were receiving now. We politely requested our promised rations and suggested that fruit, *quallies* (a metal circular cooking utensil used to cook rice and prepare hot drinks) and further medical supplies would also be appreciated. We finished our letter with an assurance that the men could work to the satisfaction of Nippon Tsun if given adequate food and medical supplies.

Our efforts were in vain: we received no reply. I do, however, feel compelled to acknowledge that Lieutenant Watanabe did seem to be genuinely concerned about our wellbeing — when any of our men were beaten by Nippon Tsun employees he would attempt to investigate the incident and reprimand the guilty party. The fact that he did not respond to our written request was more than likely due to an authority higher than him, and that Nippon Tsun had absolutely no interest in humanitarian obligations. As an example of the meanness of this company, there was an occasion when the men worked from early in the morning right throughout the night. A meal was provided at midnight but this was at the expense of the next day's lunch, which the company refused to supply.

By the middle of October we were transferred to our new billets: a rice storehouse located opposite a sake factory. While we had been POWs for more than two and a half years this was the first time we had ever been enclosed in a compound. On the Railway, the jungle had acted as an impenetrable wall, but now we had the real thing: a tall wooden fence decorated with barbed wire. We were formally 'imprisoned'.

I slept in a small enclosure with the four British officers; our room served as sleeping quarters, an office and eating area. The men were crowded into nearby billets which consisted of two floors, one on the ground, the other about two metres above it; with the upper floor reached by vertical ladders. Lighting, both natural and artificial, was very poor and after our distressing journey in the dark hold of the *Kibitsu Maru* none of the men appreciated feeling so confined again.

Cooking was initially done in a temporary outdoor shelter, essentially a little roof on stilts. The POW cooks had to wear overcoats while they worked in the cold, the icy air reddening their noses and cheeks. The emptying of the latrine sump was very irregular and often excrement and urine overflowed. Washing facilities were almost non-existent, with only one cold-water tap provided for close to 300 men.

The two Japanese civilian doctors continued to visit our camp weekly. They conferred with Jim Roulston and me as medical colleagues and allowed us to accept full responsibility for treatment of our own men. Nippon Tsun also employed a civilian medical orderly, Yuzo Matsumoto, a middle-aged man with a grossly deformed leg believed to be due to childhood polio. He carried his bad leg, bent at the knee, in front of his body when he walked. His voice was warm and soft and his smile broad. Matsumoto did his utmost to provide the medical supplies we needed and requested, and he frequently shared his lunch, a *binto* box of rice, fish and vegetables, with POW patients. His acts of kindness were small but involved great personal risk. He was the first Japanese man I considered a friend.

Among the 29 Australians in Sakata were seven men from the 2/10th Field Regiment and seven from the 2/15th Field Regiment, all of whom had been in Anderson Force with me in

Burma. We formed a very close-knit group. I was particularly close to Kitch Loughnan, a tall and gangly 'bushie' from Mitchell in south-west Queensland. Kitch was the youngest son of a large Irish family and he often told me stories about his life on the land where the homestead 'paddock', as he called it, consisted of a mere 24,000 hectares. Kitch had an indefatigable sense of humour and could see the positive in the bleakest of situations. I was fascinated by Kitch, along with other bushies in our group. Bushies were a breed of their own; they had a natural instinct to think 'big', possibly as a result of the way they lived their lives — on enormous properties with enormous flocks of sheep and herds of cattle. In captivity, I believe this gave them the ability to look beyond the immediate; to see each day as a single pixel in a much larger and brighter picture, which would one day end in our release. They were joyful and inspiring companions.

The days crawled by, becoming colder, as we worked for longer. At the end of the month our group of Australians was shattered when Jimmy Mullens — the energetic lifesaver from Manly — died of amoebic dysentery, a condition that causes severe diarrhoea containing a lot of mucus (bowel lining) as well as blood. He was only 23 years old. Jim was cremated at the local crematorium and his ashes were kept in a box in our camp until the end of the war.

In the following weeks four more of our men were transferred to Tokyo Hospital, also suffering amoebic dysentery. After surviving the Railway and being shipwrecked at sea it seemed incomprehensible that some of our men should now lose their lives to conditions that could so easily have been treated with the appropriate medicine. Matsumoto and the visiting doctors did their best to supply us with everything they could but emetine, used to treat amoebic dysentery, was always hard to come by. Tragically, for Jimmy Mullens, we received supplies of emetine two months after his death. We were incensed by the unnecessary waste of such bright young lives.

FOLLOWING THE LOSS OF Jimmy Mullens, bouts of despondency became far more common within our group. Our darker mood was further compounded by the official onset of winter — reportedly the coldest on record in Japan in 70 years. By the time snow fell for the first time towards the end of November, we had each been issued with a total of six blankets and a quilt, but we were still miserably cold. During the night we rolled ourselves up in our blankets to form an improvised sleeping bag, the feet of taller men almost poking out at the end.

Having never experienced snow before I had always imagined it would be a great pleasure to see soft white flakes drifting down from the sky. I recalled glossy calendars and travel brochures I had seen before the war and the memory of these images prepared me for a dazzling white landscape, but the snow in Sakata was delivered in the wake of gale force winds. The cold ran right through our bones, and frozen body joints made the slightest of movements both difficult and painful. The nights felt endless. Owing to a diet severely lacking in protein and fat we all had a frequent need to urinate. We dreaded the miserable trek from our billets to the latrine, sloshing in the icy mud, particularly when the blizzards were howling straight across from Siberia. Some of the men, especially those on the upper level of the billets, took an empty can to bed to avoid having to leave their blankets. Sometimes the cans overflowed or were knocked over to the indignant displeasure of those trying to sleep on the lower deck. (The practice was forbidden and the guilty were soon identified and dealt with by their peers.)

As winter wore on the men were soon suffering from chills, pneumonia and recurrent malaria. The billets were extremely draughty, the inside temperature frequently falling to 38 degrees Fahrenheit (three degrees Celsius) for extended periods; ice lined the windows and doorways. Winter also brought body lice, particularly among the British whose hygiene remained poorer than poor. The lice caused intolerable itching, and scratching led to infected sores on the men's rice-paper skin. During the day you could see the overcoats of men shimmering with lice beneath the sun.

Each day the men limped several kilometres through snow in their ill-fitting boots to worksites. Following numerous requests from the officers for new boots, Nippon Tsun, in all its generosity, supplied us with straw and told us to make our own. We layered the straw to form a sole and then tied them to our feet with string. As soon as we stepped in the snow the straw became wet and disintegrated. Most men spent the rest of winter working with wet and septic feet.

One of my most disturbing memories of this winter was the desperation that led to some men deliberately inducing illness in an attempt to escape labour. Back in Tavoy, when we had first started eating salt purchased from Burmese traders, we had seen several cases of gross leg oedema (today known as salt retention), which is also a sign of beriberi. All men were well aware of the side effects of salt retention, especially in salt-starved bodies such as their own. Men working in a chemical factory for Nippon Tsun had access to crude salt and, armed with the knowledge that the Japanese viewed beriberi as serious enough to warrant days in bed, some dissolved a dessert spoonful of salt in half a litre of water and drank it. Within half an hour of consuming this mixture their ankles had puffed right up. I was immediately suspicious that these sudden cases of oedema had all occurred in men from the same work group; Jim and I quickly guessed what they were up to. We rested the men and privately reprimanded them for their actions, explaining that there was a very real risk their hearts would be affected by the salt. Along with the other officers in camp, I conducted searches for salt and we made it clear to our men that this practice was entirely forbidden and extremely dangerous. Sadly, there were some we must not have convinced, and they were such deft thieves that we failed in our mission to find their contraband supplies. Two Australians and three Brits lost their young lives to cardiac beriberi during the winter as a result of their own self-destructive actions. Perhaps, in their minds, the odds of surviving a winter of labour in Sakata seemed so bad they were willing to take their chances.

Spirits lifted on Christmas Eve when we received Red Cross food parcels. The British had been given one per seven men before leaving Thailand but for the Australians this was our first since entering captivity. It was a great treat and one we decided to spread over a few days, allowing ourselves a small ration each day. The practice of 'saving the best until last' and stretching out food for as long as possible came naturally to men who had grown up during the Depression. I can still recall my father bringing home his modest pay packet each Friday night and my mother sending me down to the corner shop to buy a quarter pound (125 grams) of butter. My mother rationed this supply prudently each day to ensure it lasted for the entire week. Similar memories were commonplace among many of my mates. Along the Railway, I remember once receiving a tin of oatmeal, the genuine article, stolen from a Japanese storehouse. John Shaw and I had mixed the oatmeal with ground rice and, with careful economy, we had been able to make it last for much more than a week. Having something special to look forward to each day was possibly more of a treat than the taste of the food itself. I thought of John Shaw and my parents as I ate each item from my parcel. Our Christmas goodies included barley and beans as well as chocolate! Initially the legumes proved disastrous to the hair-trigger mechanism with which our bowels had been operating since the Railway. We were in such terrible condition our bodies just could not cope with the smallest of changes.

Lieutenant Watanabe organised some civilians to provide a piano and other musical instruments for a party on Christmas night. A tree was decorated and a stage was built in the billet. It was amazing to see how many pianists and other musicians and singers we had amongst us. Even the Japanese put on some items which we politely and quietly applauded. Several civilians attended the gathering with their children, including the two doctors who visited our camp each week. One of my most vivid memories of the party is of watching our men sharing their precious food parcels with the Japanese children as well as some of the civilians who had been kind to them. I gave the son of one of our doctors a piece of chocolate. He was completely overcome; he had never tasted it before. The look of wonderment on his face, his lips forming a wide grin of delight, is an image that has stayed with me.

Some might wonder how we could possibly interact socially with Japanese civilians after experiencing so much suffering at the hands of their nation. The distinction for me was simple. As prisoners, we were still capable of recognising that kindness was not a trait exclusive to our own kind, but rather a quality that could be found in any fellow human being. Empathy is equally universal. We could see that many of these children and civilians had also suffered immensely — losing loved ones and living on very short rations. Perhaps in the process of offering gifts to the little ones the men were thinking of their own children, siblings and relatives back home. Most of us followed a simple philosophy of 'do unto others as you would be done by' — and when civilians were caring towards us we returned the sentiment, from one human to another. Such moments were genuinely happy and heart-warming, and reminded us of the world we used to live in back home.

One of the biggest hearted Japanese civilians we encountered was a butcher named Chukichi Takahashi, a friend of Matsumoto. A stocky, good-humoured man in his 40s, I can still recall his energetic laugh which seemed to resonate from the very bottom of his belly. Takahashi was in charge of the town abattoir and responsible for the supply of meat to retail butchers in Sakata. Whenever a horse fell and broke its leg on the icy roads during the winter it was dragged on a sledge to Takahashi to be slaughtered and cut into four quarters: one quarter to be given to each of the four main meat retail outlets. The Japanese detailed three Australians to assist Takahashi: Kitch, his friend Lindsay Savage (also a cattleman) and 'Butch' Hall, a butcher by trade. Takahashi would dress the carcase and section it transversely through the ribs, and then section it again — leaving a circle of two ribs, which he rapidly concealed beneath his bench. He then sectioned the two halves vertically to create four quarters which he duly gave to the four waiting shopkeepers. When his satisfied customers left, the kindly butcher cooked a little of the forbidden meat and fed Kitch, Lindsay and Butch. With Takahashi's blessing, these three men then smuggled the remainder back into camp for the benefit of the patients in hospital. Like Matsumoto, Takahashi was prepared to take enormous personal risks to help us; it was not surprising that these two benevolent men were such good friends.

Looking back now, I still find it intriguing how quickly one's sense of right and wrong could change. In what other situation, I wonder, would we have considered it acceptable to eat horse meat, among other things? Back in September, while waiting in a holding camp just prior to embarking for Japan on the *Rakuyo Maru*, there was a near riot when our boys discovered that some of the Eurasian Dutch POWs had killed and eaten our camp's pet dog. Only months later, in the middle of winter in Sakata, the Japanese decreed that dogs were eating too much precious food and that their skins were needed for leather. The IJA ordered that all dogs be rounded up at the abattoir and slaughtered. The skins were removed and Takahashi gave the unwanted carcases to his POW assistants. Kitch, Lindsay and Butch brought the carcases back to camp and buried them beneath a pile of snow adjacent to our cookhouse. Each day the cooks removed a few dogs from the 'deep freeze' to be used in a stew. The bushies were at first horrified at the prospect of eating an animal they regarded as their best friend back home, but they quickly overcame their aversion when the stews were acclaimed by the troops. I remember experiencing great shame and revulsion on my first mouthful, but starvation of any form of protein quickly enabled me to rationalise my behaviour. Circumstances can change one's sensitivities dramatically.

APRIL WAS A MONTH of new beginnings. On the 15th the IJA assumed greater control of the camp and replaced all Nippon Tsun employees with their own troops. Our men were to continue to labour for Nippon Tsun during the day but would remain under the guard of the IJA. None of us knew why this happened — I have long suspected it was thanks to the influence of Lieutenant Watanabe — but regardless we welcomed the return of the troops in preference to the men of Nippon Tsun, who had shown no regard for whether we lived or died throughout an insufferable winter. In the changeover, I was particularly saddened to lose our civilian medical orderly, Matsumoto. Before departing he made a speech of sorrow at having to leave us and mentioned that he could be contacted through Takahashi the butcher. As he was leaving, he took me aside and with great sincerity said: 'I will miss you, very brave man.' He then handed me a small gift of a beautiful Japanese notebook, properly bound and with pages ruled into tiny squares. Matsumoto had often seen me writing in my own unbound notebook and had previously brought me a needle and thread so I could stitch it together (I was still holding true to my vow never to keep another personal diary, but I couldn't resist the urge to log dates and locations, facts and figures and a list of full details of the Australians in Sakata).

'This one much better,' Matsumoto had said to me, pointing to his gift. I knew then that I would see my friend again after the war; I would make sure of it. I have always treasured this handsome notebook and still have it in my possession to this day.

By the end of the month the remnants of winter peeled away to reveal a wondrous spring. The skies turned a cloudless baby blue and the sun shone. Throughout winter we had been surviving one day at a time, living aimlessly in some kind of foggy stupor. Now, as the days became warmer I could feel my mind slowly thawing. After making it through a horrendous winter and enduring ill treatment by Nippon Tsun, many of us returned to being incorrigible optimists. The change in season brought about a fundamental change in our attitude; we shifted from merely coping to taking responsibility for injecting new meaning into our lives. It is difficult to convey the emotional transition involved in moving from an incredibly low state of mind to such a reawakening. I recall considering how long my own luck had held and then experiencing a sudden sense of immortality; it was a premonition, of sorts, that I would make it home. Our rehabilitated optimism was further enhanced by snippets of news, courtesy of Takahashi, that Allied forces were gaining momentum.

With fresh enthusiasm I helped with the planning of a vegetable garden outside the camp. As well as supplying much needed food, it had the added advantage of providing light work for those who were too sick to work outside the camp but not sick enough — by Nippon Tsun standards — to escape labour. By this time Lieutenant Watanabe had been replaced by an equally sympathetic commander, Lieutenant Mori, and he allowed us to allocate 40 men to tend to the garden on a permanent basis. This variation of work duties more than likely saved the lives of these chronically ill men.

On Mother's Day, most appropriately, I received a telegram from my mother — the first message from home I had been given since arriving in Japan. The absence of mail from home throughout our time in captivity was an added cruelty. A word from loved ones could raise our hopes higher than any other remedy, which was possibly why our keepers rarely delivered our messages. I can still picture the pure joy on the faces of men who were lucky enough to receive a letter or Red Cross card; smiles bursting as they read news from their families, despite the fact that it was usually at least two years' old by they time they received it.

Before Christmas, I had been permitted to send a wireless message home.

> *Cheerio Mother. Christmas greetings to all relations and friends. My thoughts are with you all especially now.*
>
> *My health is good and my spirits high.*
>
> *I was delighted to receive a letter from Mother, Father, Frank and Linda and am expecting more.*
>
> *We recently arrived in Japan and are preparing for a cold snowy winter.*
>
> *We have warm clothing and blankets and the billets are comfortable.*
>
> *The food is wholesome and fruit is available . . .*
>
> *Love to all & Toosday[2]*
>
> *Rowley Richards.*

Mother's return telegram read:

> *OC 15414 NX70273 Captain C R B Richards 1912 Tokyo Camp*
>
> *Rowley received wonderful radio message. All well relieved; good luck.*
>
> *Mother Richards*

It is beyond me even now to put into words just how wonderful it was to know that my wireless message had been received — that my family knew I was alive and well and would be waiting for me on my return home.

DURING THE END OF May and the beginning of June we lost three of our older Australians for whom the winter was just too much. Out of 45 cases of pneumonia in Sakata we lost nine men; we had no suitable sulpha drugs available to treat them. In their debilitated state the men had little resistance to ward off or withstand infection.

Kitch also developed pneumonia and I took the desperate measure of attempting auto-haemotherapy, a procedure used in the Dark Ages (before chemotherapy) which I recalled from my university textbooks. With the help of Jim Roulston, I took blood from a vein in Kitch's arm and injected it into his buttock muscle. The object was to set up a reaction to stimulate the production of white blood cells which would, in turn, attack the pneumonia germs and produce a 'crisis' of high temperature and heavy sweating. The event of 'crisis' occurred in the natural course of the disease in those who survived. Kitch had been a true friend to me in Sakata, especially when I had been ill with severe diarrhoea during the worst of the winter. On occasions he had carried me like a baby through falling snow to the latrine. I would have tried anything to save his life.

I stayed by Kitch's bedside for two days following the procedure. Near unconscious he lay like a limp sack of bones on his hospital bed. He slept with his mouth slightly open, coughing and gasping. I was not well myself and Jim frequently stopped by to persuade me to go to bed, but I shook my head at him vehemently. If something had happened to Kitch and I wasn't there I would never have forgiven myself. Finally, on day three, Kitch entered the 'crisis' phase of pneumonia. I had never been so pleased to see a man's temperature skyrocket. I knew he would make it — although whether this was because of, or in spite of, our experimental treatment I cannot say. As he pulled through his crisis, steadily rallying, he became increasingly alert and I will forever remember the moment he raised his head and said, 'Thanks, Doc.'

Later that afternoon, still by Kitch's side, my attention was drawn to two Australians and a Brit waiting for me inside the hospital's examination room. With Kitch on the mend, I made my way towards them. One of the Australians, Tom Moxham, had been suffering from malaria and diarrhoea while the other, Stan Manning, had an abscess on one of his thighs, and the Brit, McFarlane, had been off colour for a day suffering a general malaise. After incising Stan's abscess I took the opportunity to closely examine the Brit's skin. I noticed a crop of vesicles (blisters) on his scalp and immediately called Jim to confirm my diagnosis of smallpox. The vesicles in smallpox appear mainly on the face, scalp, forearms and shins and are easy to recognise — I had also seen cases of smallpox on the Railway. The germs are spread by droplets from the breath and by direct contact with pustules which develop from the blisters. It seemed likely that some of us standing in the examination room would also soon be diagnosed with the viral disease.

Jim and I reported the smallpox case to Lieutenant Mori who called upon a Japanese medical officer to confirm our diagnosis. The entire camp was immediately quarantined and smallpox achieved what we had been unable to in all our time in captivity: the opportunity to give all men a complete rest for two weeks.

CHAPTER EIGHTEEN

LIBERATION AT LAST
July–September 1945

Tom Moxham, Stan Manning and I quickly followed the British lad, McFarlane, in being officially diagnosed with smallpox. In addition to the entire camp being quarantined, the four of us were placed in isolation in an unused guardhouse, where we were soon joined by four other men suffering severe dysentery. Despite feeling lousy, I was well pleased with the position of our lodgings. Located next to the main gates of the camp, right on the edge of the parade ground, the hut featured a large open doorway at the front — giving us front-row seats for keeping tabs on the guards. To the rear was a window which opened directly onto the men's latrine, providing a perfect opportunity for us to communicate with the rest of our men. Inside, conditions were cramped; there was just enough room for the eight of us to unroll our sleeping mats and stretch out full length. Initially I suffered headache, backache, shivering and loss of appetite. One of my blisters had a bleeding spot at the base, a sign I knew could indicate a fatal outcome. Most of my head and limbs were covered in red blotches and blisters that were itchy and tender. If we did not work out some way to occupy our minds in this little coop with a view, we would all readily become despondent.

Most of us had learned that a busy mind was often the only place in which we could take refuge. And after years in captivity I had come to realise that my own odds of survival had possibly been a little higher than that of many others for the simple reason that I had not only been kept busy with work, but had also had the advantage of retaining my vocation: in action, I was a doctor; in captivity, I remained a doctor. In comparison, most of the other men, aside from the padres and some of the officers, had been forced to adapt from being soldiers in action to becoming slave labourers in captivity — one hell of a leap. They had to endure sweltering days of punishing work under the brutal watch of Japanese guards. Every aspect of their working day reminded them that they were oppressed men. I considered myself blessed to be a doctor. By vocation alone I had always felt compelled to survive in order to keep helping others.

But now, stuck in the isolation hut, for the very first time in captivity I found myself denied the opportunity to perform my role as medical officer. After six days of feeling decidedly ill, I began to gather strength, as did most of the others. Many of my older vesicles started to dry up, including my bleeding spot. New blisters were still developing but our outlook did not appear to be so grim. I knew that not having a job to cling to would destroy my spirit, at the very least, so I decided to create a new purpose for my life: to keep active the minds of my fellow patients, as well as my own.

I established two main means of easing our boredom: first, detailing each of the men to prepare and give a daily talk on some part of his life and, second, keeping up with the latest news and rumours.

Each morning I allocated a topic for one of the men to talk about. For example, I remember Moxham, a country boy, speaking about bushfires; Manning, a self-taught assayer, telling us about gold mining in Victoria; a Scottish lad recounting his first train trip when he joined the Army; a Brit speaking about his local village which specialised in espalier fruit trees; and another Brit recalling his Christmas visits to his grandparents at a village 30 kilometres from his home. Seemingly everyday parts of our own lives were fascinating to others, and these sessions gave each of us the opportunity to use our imaginations; to share nostalgic and mind-nourishing memories. I spoke about everything from my riding days in Kyogle and my parents' deaf community in Sydney to anatomy dissections and artillery surveying. When talking about our respective homelands, the Brits had difficulty in comprehending the wide open spaces in Australia just as we had trouble understanding their lack of travel beyond their own small villages. We passed hour after hour listening to, and learning from, the experiences of each other.

In the evenings, keeping track of the latest news and rumours was almost a full-time job. The rest of our men in camp had returned to work after two weeks of rest and, from thereon, every day they smuggled into camp a stolen Japanese newspaper and passed it to me through the rear window of our hut. Back in Burma, our interpreter, Bill Drower, had given me lessons in reading Katakana — an angular form of Japanese characters mainly used for writing words of foreign origin. While my skills were quite rudimentary I was usually able to decipher headlines. Each night I sat cross-legged on my mat and pored over the news pages, translating out loud to my fellow patients. The eight of us would then consider these headlines in light of the various rumours men had brought back to camp from their worksites (some courtesy of Takahashi, the butcher). We sifted the plausible items from the ridiculous and the most likely version of events was then issued as a 'verbal bulletin' from our back window to the men in the latrines, who passed word to the rest of the camp. The men gobbled up our daily dispatches with delight. In captivity, information was always at a premium: what every man wanted more than anything else was a sign that the end might be in sight.

As well as the newspaper, the men also dropped off tins of meat, fish and fruit stolen from their worksites. Knowing that the guards were unlikely to search the isolation hut the men passed their heist through our rear window and asked us to hide it in return for a small cut. Two of us lifted one man on our shoulders so he could poke his head and scrawny arms through the manhole in the centre of the bamboo ceiling to secrete or retrieve the tins. Meanwhile, the other five patients stood at the windows to keep a lookout for guards. I was genuinely worried that the fragile cavity in our ceiling might cave in with the weight of the cans; it was a dicey experiment and one we were at great pains to conceal from our keepers. As news of the war became more and more positive for us we were not so keen on taking risks. Previously, risks had always seemed worthwhile — after all, we didn't feel as though we had much to lose. But now, with Allied forces making gains every day, we were even more determined to stay alive and, what's more, we had no idea how the guards might react to our misdemeanours now that the tide of the war was turning.

The vesicles on McFarlane, Manning and me cleared up by early July but we had to remain in isolation because Moxham kept developing new batches. We were overjoyed to be stuck in our little hut where we had access to food, news and could rest quite peacefully. With our established routine of preparing talks during the mornings, delivering talks in the afternoon and keeping up with the news during the evenings, the days passed quickly. By the end of the month we looked out from our front door to see the endless streams of vapour trails of large Allied bombers flying overhead, presumably to attack towns or cities to our north. It seemed that Allied forces were *seriously* closing in. We were growing quietly confident that the war might soon be over.

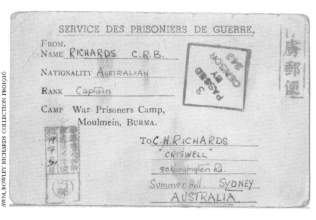

LEFT I addressed this postcard home to: 'CRISWELL'. I was hoping that if my parents ever received the card they would recognise my intended message: that Charles Richards (my 'proper' name) IS WELL. The card did in fact make it home and my parents instantly understood my message.

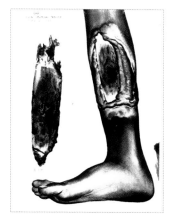

LEFT An illustration of a tropical ulcer typical of those our men suffered along the Railway. Treating the ulcers was a painstaking and time-consuming process. Gouging or scraping the ulcers was strictly forbidden to ensure we did not damage new pink granulating tissue.

BELOW An emaciated cholera patient. The highly infectious cholera was the most feared disease along the Railway. Death from severe dehydration could result in a shockingly short period of time, just a few hours.

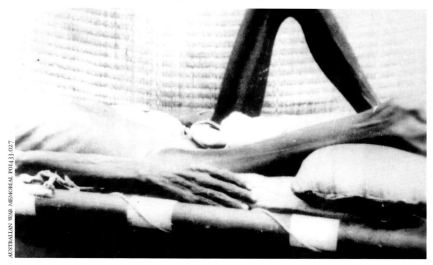

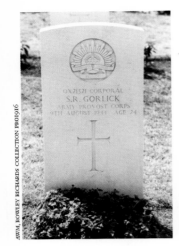

LEFT The final resting place of Corporal Gorlick, Kranji War Cemetery, Singapore. My buried diary summary and medical records were recovered from his grave several months after Corporal Gorlick's remains had been relocated.

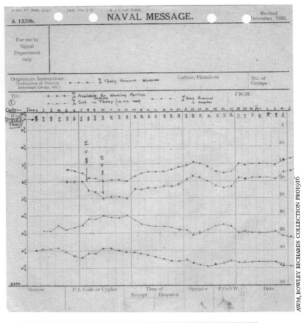

RIGHT A sample of the graphs I kept at Tavoy on Royal Navy message forms. They show the date, camp strength (top line pink); percentage available for work (bottom line pink); sick — light duty, no duty, hospital (top black line); and percentage in hospital (bottom row black).

ABOVE A sample of my record of admissions to hospital huts at Tavoy from 29 May 1942, showing diagnosis, date of onset, date of admission, date of discharge, nationality, rank, name, number, age and unit.

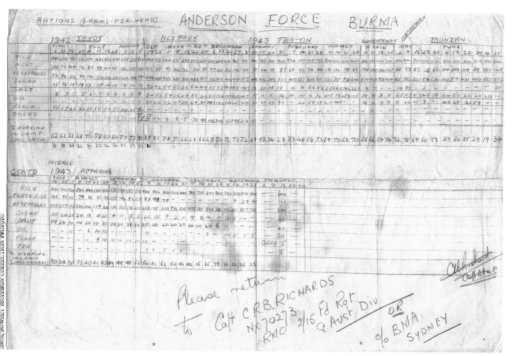

ABOVE Table showing 'A' Force camp locations, date, rations (grams per man) of rice, meat, vegetables, sugar, salt, oil, flour, bread and tea, and percentage of men working, including on camp duties (*kakaris*). This table was buried with my diary summary on Jeep Island and returned to me in 1947.

BELOW The above table in graph form.

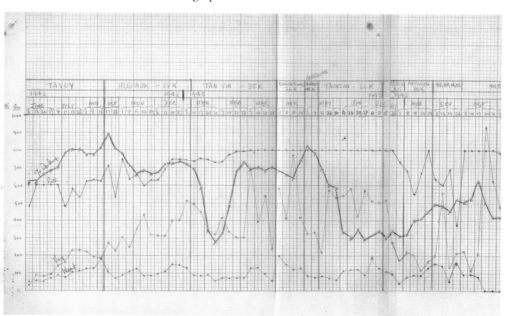

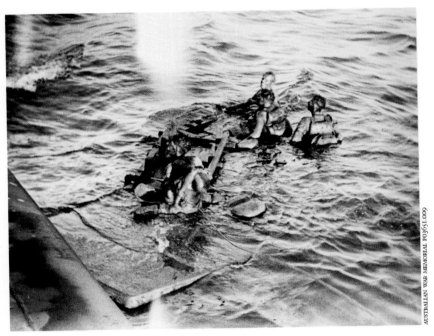

ABOVE US submarines surfaced near the site of the sinking of the *Rakuyo Maru*, where we had left behind our mates stranded on rafts. Reportedly a total of 92 Australian former POWs from the *Rakuyo Maru* were rescued and eventually made it home to relay the horrible truth about our experiences on the Railway and the torpedo attacks.

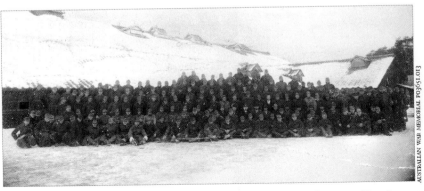

ABOVE This photo was taken by the Japanese in Sakata on Christmas Day in 1944. The winter we spent in Sakata was said to be the coldest on record in Japan in 70 years.

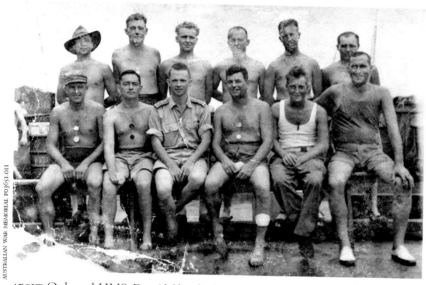

ABOVE Onboard HMS *Formidable* which carried 1,000 of us from Manila home to Australia. You can see my hair (front row, third from left) had started to grow back after being cut very short while I had smallpox. I remember I was busily trying to comb it when the ship's captain called out, 'Rowley, don't worry. Your head looks less and less like a lavatory brush every day.' (Kitch Loughnan is in the front row, far right.)

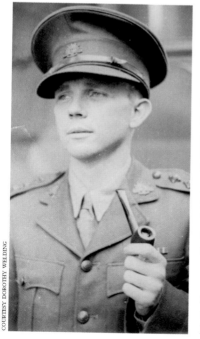

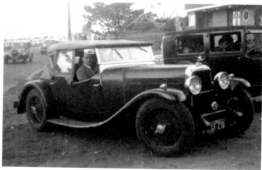

ABOVE With my deferred pay I bought my first car: a second-hand 1934 Sports Alvis Tourer Firefly convertible. It was known as 'Donald' after Donald Duck because its tail-end was slung so low to the ground.

LEFT Back home in 1945 as a returned medical captain, enjoying my first postwar Barling pipe.

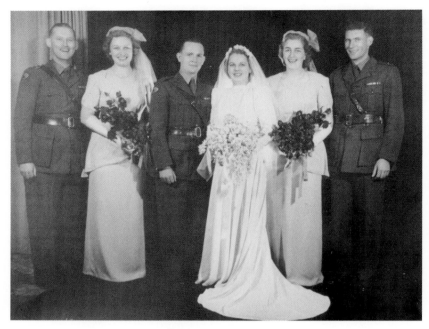

ABOVE Our wedding day. From left to right: Des Makepeace, Joan Mills, me, Beth, Bettye Mitchell and Syd Smith.

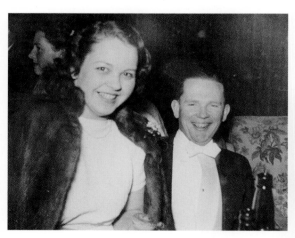

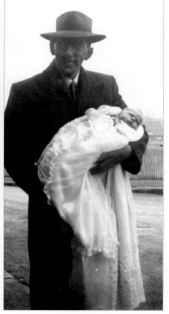

ABOVE Investing money in nightclubs, circa 1946, with Beth at Gleneagles, a popular nightclub in Potts Point.
RIGHT John Shaw was a friend for life. Here he is holding our first son, David, on his christening day.

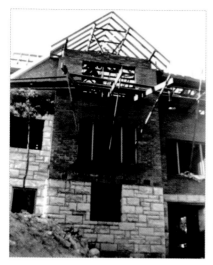

LEFT My dream home, Duart, under construction in circa 1952. This house was based on the plan John Shaw had helped me draw while in captivity in Burma. The final plan was drawn in full detail in 1949.

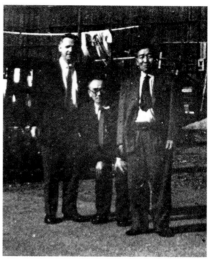

RIGHT In 1959, accompanied by Beth, I returned to Japan to visit my friends Matsumoto (centre) and Takahashi (right). I have never forgotten the kindness they showed to me and my men during our miserable winter in Sakata.

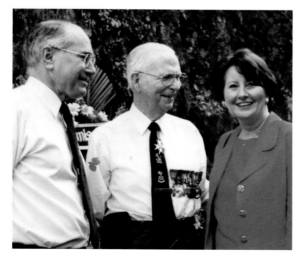

LEFT In 1998 I joined a Department of Veterans' Affairs pilgrimage to the opening of the Hellfire Pass Memorial Museum by Prime Minister John Howard and his wife, Jeanette.

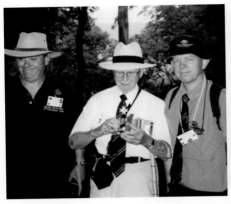

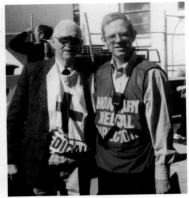

ABOVE In 2003 I returned to Thailand and Burma accompanied by my two sons, David (right) and Ian (left). I wanted to pay my final respects to my fallen comrades.

ABOVE The Sydney City to Surf Fun Run has been one of my greatest passions in life postwar. Here I am at the finish line with my son, David. In 1998, at 82 years of age, I stepped down as honorary medical director after 21 years, becoming honorary medical consultant. David, who had been my deputy, was appointed as my replacement.

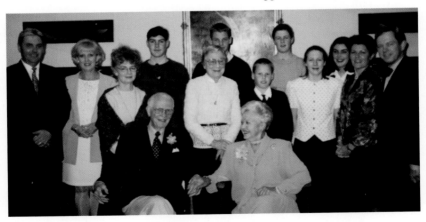

ABOVE Family photo taken at the celebration of our golden wedding anniversary, 28 June 1997. Back row (left to right): Ian and his wife Lois; Robert Raue (David's wife Maria's son); Guy (Ian's son); Charlie (David's son); Angela Raue (Maria's daughter). Middle row: Tricia Reed (family friend); Barbara Makepeace (widow of Des Makepeace); Lee (Ian's son); Belinda (David's daughter); Maria (David's wife); and David. Front row: Me and Beth, still smiling after 50 years together!

IN EARLY AUGUST THREE things happened that made us suspect the end of the war had either taken place, or was about to take place, but we would have to wait until the middle of the month for absolute confirmation of our liberation.

The first thing was a news report on 6 August. The eight of us in the isolation hut huddled around our evening newspaper, puzzled by a seemingly unbelievable front-page headline. I interpreted it as: 'One B-29 aeroplane, one bomb, Hiroshima finish.' At the time, we had no concept of atomic warfare or its shocking consequences. We speculated that Hiroshima had been bombed by Allied forces but we did not understand the devastation which had taken place — there was no picture accompanying the story. We had no idea just how radically the world of weaponry had changed during the term of our incarceration. I wondered if I had misinterpreted the words or if it was perhaps a false report, but the men had also returned to camp with rumours that Hiroshima had been destroyed. I don't remember what we talked about in the hut during that night, or what we issued in that evening's bulletin; we were obviously excited — we knew that the end really must be nigh, but at the same time we could not yet celebrate. After years of clinging to unreal deadlines ('Home by Christmas!'), we didn't dare presume our freedom was an absolute certainty. When only a few days later the headlines were similar for Nagasaki, we remained under a spell of what I would term 'cautious optimism'.

The second thing occurred on 10 August, when Sakata came in for its share of bombing. From the window of our hut we watched Allied bombers form a circle in the sky and, one by one, peel away to swoop down on a target in the harbour and then resume its position within the circle. The men returned to camp that night with first-hand accounts of how the planes had strafed the town and destroyed the Japanese anti-aircraft guns. We allowed our hopes to rise another notch. (In hindsight, it's difficult to believe we could have been so calmly philosophical about our own odds of escaping an Allied attack; I think after surviving a shipwreck one's outlook on 'chance' becomes relative — and, in relative terms, we suspected the targets would be ships, factories, anti-aircraft posts and larger buildings as opposed to our own camp. Strangely, I do not recall experiencing any real fear that we might die at the hands of our own forces.)

The third thing happened on 15 August. We had been maintaining a vigilant eye on our keepers, forever on the lookout for some kind of change in their behaviour to verify our suspicions that the war was over. On this particular afternoon we observed some guards setting up a table outside their own guardhouse. A wireless set was carried across the parade ground and placed on top of the table and the guards were soon on parade before Lieutenant Mori. The wireless was switched on and the guards yelled out 'Banzai!' repeatedly, so we knew the voice coming from the radio had to belong to someone of high standing. As the broadcast continued, the guards became increasingly subdued. We were not close enough to hear the radio but we watched as their facial expressions tightened; tears rolled down the cheeks of some.

Inside the hut, we chattered rapidly. That had to have been the voice of the Emperor advising of Japan's surrender. The war was over; it must be! We waited: surely Lieutenant Mori would soon be heading our way. But nothing happened. The guards were dismissed and, with their heads hanging low, they dispersed within the camp without another word. If Japan had surrendered, why wasn't any one telling us? We waited for the men to return from work — their rumours seemed to match our hopes, but there was no newspaper on this day to confirm what we wanted to hear.

To pass the time, I continued writing in my unbound notebook. I was still recording dates of significant events and summaries of my previous reading and thinking — especially notes on the meaning of life and other philosophical topics I had discussed with John Shaw along the Railway. These I rewrote and expanded while the events were still fresh in my mind and before the excitement of what I believed to be the end of the war caught up with me.

The next morning all men were sent to work as usual but, that afternoon, the work parties returned very early and our guards abandoned their posts. The following day the men were not sent to work and the moment we had been waiting for finally arrived during evening roll call.

Standing at the front door of our isolation hut, we watched our men standing on parade. Armed guards were positioned along the sides of the columns of our men and Lieutenant Mori walked slowly to the front. He wore tiny spectacles on the bridge of his nose and a sword hung by his side. He looked immaculate. Glancing down at a small piece of paper clasped in his hands, he read his announcement in English:

The longed for day of peace has arrived . . . you must obey your own officers . . . we are concerned for your health and your safety . . . myself, the guards and Military Police will do our best to protect you.[1]

There was no hypocrisy in Mori's announcement, which he read with great dignity and respect; no postulating over how fortunate we were to have been in the care of the IJA. I think he knew we deserved nothing but the truth.

Inside our minds, we were bursting with joy, but there was no cheering, no din of spontaneous applause, no tears of relief. We would not celebrate in the face of our enemy. Nor did the Japanese react. Both sides were silent. Many might question such a lacklustre response, but unless you have been a prisoner of war it will be difficult to understand, just as it is almost impossible for me to put such a situation into words. After years in captivity, we had become disciplined in the art of self-control — we were experts at masking emotions in front of our keepers. On the Railway, the penalty for emotional outbursts had always been physical. We had learned long ago to keep our thoughts, feelings and hopes inside our own minds; they were safe there. Surrounded by armed guards, the poker game between 'us and them' was still very much in progress. The minutes following Lieutenant Mori's speech were peaceful. For most of us it was time to acknowledge our own personal triumph over a relentless endurance test: our victory was survival. I was 29 years old and free — well, almost.

MY IMMEDIATE CONCERN WAS that eight of us were still stranded in the isolation hut (because Moxham still had blisters we were all considered contagious). We were bitterly disappointed not to be allowed out to quietly celebrate the end of the war with our closest mates. The Japanese guards remained on duty, charged with the task of protecting our camp from possible attacks by angry Japanese civilians. What an irony of fate it would have been if we had been wiped out by civilians after the war was over. The wrath of mothers and wives who had lost their menfolk surely could have done just that.

Remembrance of our deceased mates was very much on our minds. Captain Peirce conducted a memorial church service in their honour, where the individual names of all our fallen men were read aloud in between hymns and prayers. Regardless of any man's religious leanings or otherwise, everyone participated while we watched from the open doorway of our hut.

Over the next few days following the end of the war, we enjoyed receiving a marked increase in our rations, including a whole tin of M&V (meat and vegetables) and a tin of oranges each per man per day, along with an increased ration of rice. We also received Red Cross medical supplies and clothing, along with paint and paint brushes. On the roof of our billets, in huge letters, some of the men painted 'POW'. We hoped that Allied planes would notice us sooner rather than later.

As each day passed, I began to experience a gradual realisation of freedom. My mind drifted to what I might do when I returned home. I thought about the house plans I had mapped out with John Shaw and opening a medical practice in Seaforth. I thought of my parents and brother and my relatives in Kyogle. My thoughts were only of the future: I just wanted to put the past behind me, get home and get on with living the rest of my life. Perhaps this sentiment helps to explain why no one in our camp felt compelled to 'get even' with our former sentries. During captivity, one topic of conversation that had kept us determined to stay alive was the prospect of what we would do to our keepers when we won the war. There had been much bravado and grave threats of retribution yet, in the event, when we had the opportunity to become the oppressors, all such thoughts vanished. As prisoners of war, boasting of how our guards might meet their end had helped maintain morale but it became meaningless as soon as the war was over. I think most men knew that abandoning their own sense of morality in exchange for revenge would in no way compensate for our loss of mates or the incomprehensible suffering. No one had the right to treat a fellow human being as we had had been treated — not even us.

I remember one occasion, a couple of weeks following Japan's surrender, when a drunken Japanese officer staggered up to one of our men, drew his sword and shouted, '*Banzai!*' Our man, armed with a fixed bayonet rifle, simply reversed arms and knocked the Japanese officer to the ground. The officer picked himself up and beat a hasty retreat. Another Australian standing nearby asked our lad why he hadn't run the bastard through with his bayonet. He simply replied: 'If I did that, I would be no better than those I despise.' The hatred and anger was still very, very raw but there was an honourable determination not to resort to the same callous conduct to which we had been subjected. I have heard and read that in other camps reprisals did take place and, if they did, I could neither condone nor condemn such behaviour. Captivity and torture affect men in very different ways.

IT WAS THE END of August, on the morning we were due to be released from the isolation hut, when our ears suddenly pricked: the humming of planes in the distance heralded the arrival of two magnificent American B-17s. The eight of us ran from the hut, waving our lean arms hysterically at the low-flying aircrafts. Light on our feet, we leapt in the air like excited young boys as we watched 44-gallon drums, tied to parachutes, tumble from the hollow bellies of the planes and then plummet to the ground (many of the parachutes failed to open). Without a Japanese guard in sight I felt free, at least momentarily, to cut loose and celebrate with unmistakeable pleasure. After years of talking in measured sentences the eight of us screamed our lungs out.

The drums landed about 100 metres south of the camp, bursting open on impact. Food littered the ground — tinned fruit, soup, milk, cocoa, sugar, fruit juice, bean powder and bouillon powder, chewing gum and American chocolate. Attached to one of the items of food was a note:

ALLIED PRISONERS

The Japanese Govt has surrendered. You will be evacuated by Allied Nations forces as soon as possible. Until that time your present supplies will be augmented by air drops of U.S. food, clothing & medicines. The first drop of these items will arrive within one hour or two hours. Clothing will be dropped in standard packs for units of 50 or 500 men. Bundle markings, contents & allowances per man are as follows:-

Drawers 2, Undershirt 2, Sox pair 2, Shirt 1, Trousers 1, Jacket field 1, Belt, web, waist 1, Cap H BT 1, Shoes, pair 1,

Handkerchiefs 3, Towel 1, Laces, shoe 1, Kit, sewing 1, Soap, toilet 1, Razor 1, Blades, razor 1, Brush, tooth 1, Paste, tooth 1, Comb 1, Shaving cream 1, Insecticide 1.

There will be instructions with food & medicines for use & distribution.

Caution: Do not overeat or over-medicate. Follow directions.[2]

In my unbound notebook I recorded this event as 'the thrill of a lifetime'; upon reflection, that was a *gross* understatement! Perhaps I had run out of words or was just too elated to spend time putting down my true responses on paper because, looking back now, I remember feeling as though I was moving towards a profound sense of happiness, into a state of mind where I would be free to enjoy the pleasure of living in peace again.

ALL IN ALL, WE had to wait about a month from the end of the war until we could depart for Australia. While we were restless to get out of Sakata as fast as possible, we were also determined to maintain morale and discipline to the very end. The Japanese gave us a radio so we could keep up to date with Allied broadcasts about our impending evacuation. We just had to be patient.

Captain Barrett and I worked on the preparation of nominal rolls, details of the deceased, rates of sickness, food, and specific notes about our treatment by Nippon Tsun. Our records were to be presented as a combined report signed by all five officers of the Sakata camp. There was a lot of paperwork to be done. It was imperative for me to detail the facts; further evidence to complement my diary summary and records still buried on Jeep Island. While I wanted to move on with the rest of my life, I did not want the history of our group to pass unrecorded or any of our lost mates to be forgotten. I hoped my writings might one day be used in war crimes proceedings.

The following weeks were filled with celebrations and cheer. Released from isolation, I was enormously pleased to be reunited with Kitch and my other Australian mates. Kitch was one of the first to welcome me back into 'society' and was proud to tell me how well he had recovered from pneumonia. With the assistance of Lieutenant Mori, we managed to obtain sewing machines and bolts of coloured silk to make our homeland flags. Each of the nationalities — British, Australian, as well as American and Dutch (who had stopped off on their way to other POW camps further north) — conducted frantic working bees. Among the Australians there was great debate over the number of points on each star — five or seven? How many stars did we need in total and how they should be aligned? Should the Southern Cross sit vertically or be tilted to one side? The Yanks were having even more trouble — 50 stars and a lot of stripes were posing all sorts of problems for men who were not well trained in the craft of sewing. While our men were at it, they made stripes for the NCOs and pips for the officers. I wore my new cloth pips with indescribable pride. The military police, who had been attached to our camp to protect us, patrolled outside while the Japanese flag was lowered and our flags were raised on tall timber poles. Two hundred and ninety-two former prisoners of war, now free men, saluted their respective flags in a moving ceremony that marked the official changing of the guard. Our own men were then charged with the duty of protecting our camp. The Japanese officers marched their guards off parade and dismissed them — permanently.

We were invited to various receptions and celebrations (even one hosted by Nippon Tsun). The Japanese attempted to atone for their past with lavish dinners held in posh restaurants. We did not see any point in rejecting their offers; the war was over and they had their own problems just as we had ours, but aside from the few civilians who had been kind to us, we were filled with unspoken animosity towards them. While these men were not in the same class as the Railway guards, we would never forget nor forgive the individuals responsible for our treatment throughout the bitter winter in Sakata.

One of my fondest memories of this 'in between' time was meeting another Japanese civilian, Mrs Narita. I was in town with Kitch buying a few trinkets to take home when we were approached by a refined middle-aged Japanese woman who spoke excellent English. She had a pale face and wore a traditional kimono; her dark hair was swept back into a tidy bun. She introduced herself and told us her husband had been in the Japanese Legation in London for 30 years;[3] she felt very sympathetic to the Brits and, by extension, us. She was insistent on helping us and took Kitch and me to a silk shop, where I bought a kimono, an *obi*, a bag and a few other bits and pieces for my family. A few days later we ran into Mrs Narita again in Sakata and she asked if she could show us a special place. The kindly woman took Kitch and me, as well as Jim Roulston and a few others, to Honmer's Garden — a charming Japanese garden featuring small arched bridges over tiny running creeks, stepping stones and delicately trimmed miniature shrubs and trees. I will never forget the sense of tranquillity we experienced inside this garden. A large and quiet landscape had been created in the smallest of spaces. Rocks seemed to represent mountains, tiny pools could have been lakes, and raked pebbles looked like a long shoreline. Sealed away from the rest of the city by fences and gates, it provided a solitary and scenic retreat. It seemed impossible that our ghastly living quarters had been so close to a place of such idyllic beauty.

Thanks to ongoing food drops and increased rations, we fattened up quite quickly; the skin of men at last becoming separated from their ribs by a layer of flesh. Most men put on at least ten kilograms in a matter of weeks. Lying in bed at night with a full stomach, my mind buzzed with thoughts of home. But my hopes for the future were also accompanied by anxiety about whether I would ever fit in again in Australia. How would I be treated? Would I be able to father children? Would I be capable of remembering prewar social graces? Would we be reviled for surrendering during the Malayan campaign? Our bodies were on the mend, but what about our minds? There was no way of knowing the answers to my questions. All I could do was take some comfort in the thought that if I could survive captivity, surely I could face any future challenges waiting for me back home.

ON THE MORNING OF 12 September we received orders that we were to leave for Sendai, a port on the east coast of Japan, just after midnight. Finally, we were about to embark on our long journey home. Aside from my souvenirs, I had few belongings to pack, having given most of my Red Cross goodies to Matsumoto and Takahashi in appreciation of their kindness. Many of the Australians did likewise, and when we left Sakata these generous civilians found themselves relatively wealthy in terms of cigarettes, chocolate and clothing. The previous week Takahashi had presented me with a beautiful kimono. 'This is for happy occasions,' he said when handing me the neatly folded garment. 'There will be no more happy days in Japan. Please, take it.'

I placed the kimono inside my pack with the notebook Matsumoto had given me wrapped inside. Along with my medical records and writings, these two items were my most valuable possessions.

Later that same morning we commandeered one large bottle of premium sake per man, allegedly reserved for the Emperor. Each bottle arrived wrapped in fine white rice paper. After the issue of sake, Keith Martin, an Australian warrant officer, came to the officers' quarters with a message for me: 'Would you please join the men in their celebrations?'

Captain Peirce and Captain Pote-Hunt look mortified. Their faces turned pale and their eyes glared at me, as if to say: 'Surely not, Richards.'

'Love to,' I said. I joined Keith and left the jaws of these Brits gaping at the floorboards of our billet.

We drank the sake direct from the bottle, as if it was a longneck of our favourite beer. We continued drinking all afternoon, bursting into song with 'Waltzing Matilda' and other favourites until our voices were hoarse. When I returned to the officers' quarters for the evening meal I was severely chastised and sent to Coventry by my British counterparts for 'behaviour unbecoming of an officer'. One of them said: 'It's just not done, Richards: an officer drinking with his men.'

'It is by this officer,' I said, by this stage my speech was somewhat slurred.

I can only imagine that these British officers must have been feeling quite lonely, with little comfort from their own men (other than in a deferential way). I suppose they did their best in the manner in which they believed was correct — but it was very different from the Australian way. After a few choice words I returned to my men and ate with them instead. This was the final straw in my long-running battle with the regular British Army officers.

By the time we marched out of camp just after midnight, we were close to the staggering stage but managed to pull ourselves together sufficiently to march proudly, straight as chips, from the camp to Sakata's railway station, our homemade Australian flag flapping at the front of our column. We piled into the waiting train and fell into a deep and inebriated sleep.

SOME TIME LATER, I was awakened by the sound of an Australian voice, an officer from HMAS *Bataan* announcing we had arrived in Sendai. It was 13 September 1945 — exactly one year and one day since we had been torpedoed on *Rakuyo Maru*. It is not his words of comfort that I remember now but rather his tone of heartfelt sympathy: even though we had gained condition, he was visibly shocked by our still relatively gaunt bodies. For years we had been living with guards immune to our physical deterioration and we, too, had become so accustomed to looking at one another's skeletal forms that it no longer occurred to us that our appearance might affect others. To experience genuine compassion from a fellow Australian was almost too much for us to bear. Under the guise of a hangover many of us buried our emotional faces in our hands.

From Sendai, we boarded HMS *Wakeful,* a small British destroyer, which was bound for Tokyo Bay. I sat with Kitch and a group of other Australians. It was a grey, overcast day with howling winds. We were at the tail end of a typhoon. It was a rough trip; the destroyer ploughed through the waves. There was spray everywhere, washing over the deck and up to the bridge. We quickly became claustrophobic in the ward room, as well as seasick, so spent the rest of the journey out on the deck, getting wet but at least enjoying some fresh air. We still couldn't stand the feeling of being enclosed.

Perhaps there is one particular moment in everyone's life that stands out above all others. For me, at least within the chapters of my life covering the war, it was our arrival in Tokyo Bay late that same afternoon. As we sailed into the enormous harbour, we were confronted by convoys of huge ships — battleships, aircraft carriers, cruisers — of British, US and Australian origin. Kitch and I with the others in our little group ran to the edge of the railing to take a closer look. HMAS *Shropshire* and USS *Missouri,* which had taken the Japanese surrender, and others including HMS *King George V,* dressed ship: there were countless rows of men in white uniforms lining their decks and they seemed to be cheering and waving at *us.* HMAS *Shropshire* dipped her Australian flag in salute to our ship, which had also dipped its ensign. We were a few hundred metres away, too far to see the faces of these men but close enough to hear them yell out three boisterous cheers. We could not understand what the fuss was about — after all, we were only former prisoners of war who had done nothing to help win the war.

One of the ship's crew came over to us and said, 'I hope you realise, that was for all of you men.'

Still somewhat sake-stung and exhausted, I experienced a gentle sensation of unravelling; my self-control waned, allowing repressed emotions to surface, unleashed at last. I felt almost weightless: free. It is impossible to describe exactly what I felt at that moment, it eludes me even now.

I hugged Kitch, tears spilling down my face.

'By God, what a sight,' I said, trying to compose myself. Kitch's face lightened as he nodded in agreement. He couldn't speak — but that didn't matter; there would be plenty of days ahead to talk, we had all the time in the world.

Gazing at my mates around me, I wondered not so much why so many men had died in Japanese captivity, but rather how the hell so many had managed to survive. It had been a very long war. I couldn't wait to get home.

EPILOGUE

When we assembled on deck early in the morning, a fleet of small vessels was surrounding our ship. They gave us a noisy welcome all the way down the harbour to Circular Quay, horns blaring. I stared up at the magnificent bridge I had loved so much as a boy, arched over beautiful Sydney Harbour on a perfect day: the water sparkling the brightest of blues and the sun glowing high in the sky. It was 13 October 1945 and I was home at last.

A cheering crowd of hundreds, mainly officials, met us at the wharf. We were greeted by women from the Red Cross who gave each of us a white paper bag containing a packet of cigarettes, matches and sweets, and directed us towards buses. As we drove through the city, I looked out the window to see the streets lined with more and more people. I can still picture crowds throwing steamers towards us down George Street in the city and then along Parramatta Road, all the way to Ingleburn camp, where our families were waiting for us.

From the steps of the bus I scanned the thousands of figures before me, their hands waving overhead, and almost immediately spotted the heads of my father and Uncle Arthur towering above most others; my mother and Aunt Linda were standing in front of them. Tears flowed unashamedly as I hurried through the masses towards them.

'Thank God,' I remember my mother whispering, my head resting on her shoulder in our embrace. I hugged all four of them one at a time. We were elated by our reunion; never before had we been so openly familiar.

'You look good,' Uncle Arthur said, his eyes moving from my head to my toes. And I think perhaps I did indeed look well. I was nothing like what I had been even a month before. After the war had finished I had remained in Sakata for almost four weeks, plenty of time to start fattening up on increased rations. From Sakata I had spent another ten days in Manila,[1] eating continuously, and then throughout the sea voyage home there had been unlimited food. All of us had regained a lot of weight and condition, more than enough to take the edge off our formerly frightening appearance.

Arthur drove all of us back to Summer Hill, where my brother Frank and the Martins, our neighbours, were waiting for me inside our home. Ivy Martin, quite an artist, had brought a floral arrangement in my honour. In the privacy of our lounge room, it felt as though everyone wanted to talk at once, bursting with questions and stories — there was so much to say — but in reality we all remained reserved, each adult hanging back to allow another to speak. Absent at our family gathering were my grandparents. Grandfather Polson had died not long before the war and Grandmother Polson passed away just prior to my return. I have no recollection of the details of my grandmother's death, nor can I find reference to the specific date she died. (Perhaps I had experienced so much death by then I could block out this loss, too.)

Away from the crowds at Ingleburn, I had the chance to look closely at my parents. The quiet joy on their faces could not hide the terrible anxiety they had suffered. Both had aged: my mother looked tired and my father's hair had thinned. My mother told me the story of how three survivors from the *Rakuyo Maru* who had been rescued by the American submarines, had separately contacted her to say they had seen me die. The first claimed I had drowned, the second maintained I had succumbed to malaria at sea and the third told her I had gone mad with thirst.[2] It was then that I realised my family had experienced their own war. Over the past three and a half years they had lived from day to day wondering and worrying. They had not only imagined the worst but been told the worst — that I had died at sea — all the while still hoping for the best.

After a few days in Sydney with my family — and a special visit to the nuns at the Mater Hospital in North Sydney[3] — I returned to Kyogle with Arthur and Linda to meet old friends and see my young cousin Pat. When we pulled up outside the house in Arthur's car, Pat ran outside and flung her slender arms around my neck. Now seventeen years old, she had grown into a beautiful young woman. I hugged her warmly as she sobbed into my chest. I smoothed the top of her hair and she lifted her head, a wide smile breaking her tears.

'I have something for you,' I said. From my pocket I pulled out her photo, the one she had given to me before I had left. 'I carried it always,' I told her. 'It kept me safe.'

Pat took the photo from me and gave me another hug. 'I knew you would come home.'

Arthur and Linda organised a party at their house to celebrate my homecoming. At the time, rationing was still in place, and I remember friends, neighbours and patients arriving with precious remnants of alcohol they had been saving: one-fifth of a bottle of whiskey, a third of a bottle of brown muscat, a quarter of a bottle of gin, as well as supplies of dry and sweet sherry and other wines. To stretch the grog out for as long as possible, a few of us younger men, aided by Father Nichols, the local Catholic priest who was quite a character, decided to concoct a punch. We poured the dregs from all the bottles into a baby's bath we had already part filled with chopped fruit and lemonade and then mixed it all together.

Present at the party were patients of Arthur's as well as my own friends: a gathering of people from varying religions and to begin with, as usual, no one would associate with anyone outside their own faith. Before long, however, things changed. As the night progressed and more and more of the punch was consumed — most guests not realising it was alcoholic — I watched with great satisfaction as merry Catholics talked and hugged Protestants like old friends; there was friendly banter, back slapping and good humour amongst all. I was delighted.

I think after everything I had experienced at war, I returned home even less tolerant of prejudice. Everyone has a right to believe in whatever they want to believe, but I consider it the responsibility of every individual to at least try to understand the beliefs of others, recognise differences, and, above all else, respect diversity. Too many wars have been fought over religion and differing belief systems: who is anyone to say their way of life is right and another's is wrong? I may never forgive the individual Japanese men who made my life a misery in captivity, but I vowed never to apply a blanket rule that I would hate all Japanese: I have witnessed first-hand the kind of cruel behaviour hatred can produce. And I only have to remember the kindness of my two friends in Sakata, Takahashi and Matsumoto, to know that neither religion nor race have anything to do with an individual's capacity for benevolence and compassion.

Of course, the Kyogle party was only a temporary triumph. The next day every one in town, sober again, returned to their bigoted ways, walking on opposites sides of the street from one another. To this day I still cannot understand it.

BACK HOME IN KENSINGTON Road, Summer Hill, reunions remained a priority. Longing for privacy — something I had not had for years — I rented a room at a hotel in Kings Cross so I could talk with relatives of men who did not return, as well as catch up with mates I had not seen for a long time.

The night my good friend John Shaw knocked on the door of my room was one of the best. We greeted each other with a firm handshake and ear-to-ear smiles. Last time I saw John, his arms and legs were like sticks. Now, having regained condition, he was once again a fit man, the cyclist he used to be. He came inside and, while I was opening a bottle of scotch, settled himself into a chair and reached into his coat pocket.

'I believe this belongs to you, Rowley,' he said, smiling and holding a notebook in his outstretched hand. I recognised it immediately; it was Part 2 of my original diary which I had left with him for safekeeping at Tamarkan.

I took the notebook, struggling with my emotions. 'Thank you,' I managed.

John then apologised that he had been forced to jettison the bundle of letters which I had written based on my complete diary.[4] The bulk of papers had proved too much of a risk so, forced to choose, he saved my notebook, carrying it with him in the false bottom of a billycan. I couldn't have been more grateful.

We spent that evening sharing the bottle of scotch, relaying to each other what we had experienced since I had left with the Japan Party. It was a joyous evening: we didn't discuss the horrors of war or captivity. Not talking openly about the past had already become a custom to which nearly all former prisoners of war adhered, and John and I were no exception.

Days later I was reunited with Jim Armstrong. Jim, too, had regained condition. He was again a big man, but still gentle. His formerly grey hair had turned white.

'Old Silver,' I said, greeting him at my front door with an embrace.

'Baby Doctor,' he said. His voice was still soft. We spent the evening in much the same way as I had with John Shaw: catching up on news of mates and talking — in general terms only — about what had happened to each of us since we had parted ways at Tamarkan. Miraculously, Jim returned all of the medical records we had kept from Tavoy and the Railway, together with our microscope and a set of Japanese surgical instruments.

Slowly, friends and fragments from my past were turning up at home; further reminders of experiences I would carry with me for the rest of my life. Yet the biggest piece which remained missing from my puzzle was my diary summary and records, which were then still buried beneath the cross at the head of Corporal Gorlick's grave on Jeep Island.

During our journey home to Australia, when we had stopped over in Manila, I'd been interviewed by members of the War Crimes Commission to give my version of events. (As the only officer to survive the *Rakuyo Maru* sinking I came in for quite some attention.) At the time I told them how I had buried a diary summary, including medical records, and drew them a freehand map of where they might be able to find it. The War Crimes officers had promised they would contact me if they ever recovered my treasure, and I never stopped hoping that one day it would find its way back to me.

ON 7 DECEMBER I became, officially, what had been the ambition of all men while we had been in captivity: a 'returned soldier'. With my deferred pay I bought a car which became my pride and joy. It was a second-hand 1934 Sports Alvis Tourer Firefly convertible; black with grey interior. It was soon known as 'Donald', after Donald Duck because its tail-end was slung so low to the ground. I invested the remainder of my pay in shares and on catching up with friends at Prince's, Romano's, Carl Thomas and other well-known nightclubs in Sydney.

By January it was time to resume my career. I returned to St Vincent's Hospital in Darlinghurst as a Relieving Junior Resident

Medical Officer. Back at work, I felt somewhat left behind: I had arrived home to a changed medical world. There wasn't a great deal of difference in surgical procedures, but new drugs were revolutionising medical treatments. Antibiotics were being introduced and there was much for me to learn. I attended a medical refresher course at Sydney University that was held especially for veterans. Each night I buried my nose inside the covers of textbooks, absorbing as much as I could about this new world of drugs, before heading out on the town. It was a hectic period, with most former POWs trying to find a balance between working hard and playing hard, attempting to make up for stolen time.

For the first month or so back home I attended a continuous series of meetings with mates to catch up on one another's activities since we last met, but by April we were holding regular group reunions and decided to officially form the 2/15th Field Regiment Association. Postwar there was some residual antipathy from the men directed towards certain officers. Having been an RMO, I was seen as neither fish nor fowl, and was nominated and elected as president of the Association (a position I hold to this day). We focused Association activities on raising money to help comrades in need and the widows and children of our lost mates.

The mateship between former prisoners of war had only been enhanced since returning home. I resumed my close friendship with Des Makepeace, whom I had known since childhood and travelled with throughout my Militia, fighting and captivity days. We felt secure in one another's company and no other friend would ever know me so well. Ongoing friendships with former prisoners of war provided something which was lacking in our pre-war friendships, and even relationships with our closest family members: a shared history. We often agreed amongst ourselves that being an ex-Japanese prisoner of war was like being a member of *the* most exclusive club. Amongst us there has always been a mutual dependence which is understood but never stated. The fact that we knew what each other had lived through was enough. Socially, we recalled humorous incidents, mostly stories that were at the expense of the Japanese; how so and so had outwitted a certain guard or got away with sneaking out of camp to trade at night. Just as it had in captivity, the ritual of humour offered escape. If unpleasant elements of the past were raised they would be discussed in a dispassionate manner, getting whatever it was off our chests and moving on quickly. There was never the need to talk of specific suffering, nor a call to enter into personal exchanges centring on pity or sentiment. That wasn't our way; we remained crack-hardy men.

There is no doubt all of us had returned home as changed men. To some extent, many of us became more cynical — we were not the same naïve boys who had left home for the first time in July 1941, impatient to be sent into action. Psychologically, I found myself far more tolerant of human weaknesses, such as alcoholism or an honest mistake, but extremely intolerant of anyone who was conscious of their own deception, no matter how small, for example someone deliberately cheating in a game of cards. Any form of intentional wrongdoing struck a raw nerve and I could not accept it. Claustrophobia was also a condition many of us endured as a result of memories of the awful sea voyage in the dark hold of the *Kibitsu Maru*. I avoided the downstairs sections of restaurants and could not tolerate standing in a crowded lift. Physically, aside from recurring malaria and damage to my hearing, my health immediately postwar was remarkably good: I was lucky.

WOMEN HAD BEEN ABSENT from our lives for far too long and those of us who returned home as single men were keen to regain lost ground: we had already missed so much of our young adulthood. I met many women whom I liked and took out but I

was very conscious of the way some tended to consider me —
not only as a doctor (an occupation which seemed to qualify a
man as a 'good catch') but also as a returned prisoner of war: I was
often treated with what I would call embarrassing warmth, like a
homecoming hero. Something with which I was not at all
comfortable and knew would never bode well for an equal
partnership. But when I met Beth McNab, I found a very
different kind of woman.

In late July 1946 I was still a resident at St Vincent's and had
just started dating a young nurse from the dressings department,
Mignon Scantlebury, who, at that time, happened to be staying at
Beth's flat in Kings Cross. Mignon invited me to the flat for
dinner one night while Beth was at home and, during the course
of the evening, I made a faux pas that ultimately proved to be to
my own benefit.

During conversation over dinner, I passed a flippant comment
that if a patient arrived at St Vincent's casualty with a misdiagnosis
I always knew it came from a particular doctor's practice in
Darlinghurst; I held that doctor in very low regard. I was not
aware that this same doctor was the father of Mignon's former
boyfriend, for whom she obviously still had feelings. Enraged,
Mignon rose from the dinner table, cursing me, and then
disappeared into the bedroom. I had clearly been dumped.

The blow was softened by the fact that I was already quite
taken with Beth. While Mignon stayed in her room, Beth and I
remained chatting at the dinner table until quite late. Beth was
not only very attractive but an incredibly positive person who
treated me as an equal. She was 25 years old and uncommonly
independent: she had a job (as a nurse), her own apartment and a
telephone. And she wasn't one to agree to disagree; she knew how
to confront me head on, and I liked that very much. We had our
first argument that very same evening at the flat. Unaware that I
was former prisoner of war, Beth made a statement about feeling

great sympathy for former Australian prisoners of war of the Japanese. In reply, I made an off-handed crack that those men should never have surrendered but continued to fight in the Malayan campaign (which is perhaps what I subconsciously felt). Beth was incensed. 'How dare you,' I remember her saying, her face livid. 'My cousin was a POW.'

Not wanting to be turned out on the street, it was then that I confessed to Beth that I, too, had been a prisoner of war. Like most nurses, Beth had been briefed by superiors to handle prisoners of war with the utmost care; to be cautious in her inquiries, so as not to 'fire them up'. Beth later told me that from the information she had been given, she had been prepared to expect traumatised, unstable men. And there I was, an apparently perfectly 'normal' man with a very young face, claiming to have been a prisoner of war. She didn't buy that; not for a second. In fact, she called me a liar.

I asked Beth to look at the back of my head. The hair at the front of my scalp had grown back brownish but it was still very grey at the base of my neck. I explained how my head had been shaved when I had smallpox in Sakata and how it had only just grown back. (It was well known that the hair of many prisoners of war had turned grey owing to stress.) And that was how Beth learned the first piece of information about my war past — but it would take many more years together for the rest to be revealed.

By then it was quite late in the evening. Before the dinner-table drama with Mignon, I had asked both Mignon and Beth to join me at a supper club after dinner. I knew there was no longer any chance of Mignon inviting me to the flat again so I asked Beth if she would still like to go out for supper with me.

'You were Mignon's guest and you have offended her,' she said. 'I think you should leave.' And so I did, but not without intentionally leaving my pipe in her lounge room to give me a legitimate reason to return.

Days later I received a telephone call at the hospital from Beth, politely informing me I had left my pipe at her flat, just in case I was wondering where it was. Smiling to myself, I thanked her very much and invited her out for dinner. Beth declined again, maintaining she had to wash her hair or some other excuse of the same ilk, but on my third attempt she relented, finally agreeing to have dinner with me. That dinner marked the beginning of the rest of our lives together.

Beth's grandmother, a doctor's widow, had warned her 'never marry a doctor; a doctor will only ever belong to his patients'. Despite this, Beth accepted my proposal in February 1947. We were married in June the same year in a military wedding at St David's Presbyterian Church in Haberfield, the same church in which my parents had been married.[5] Des Makepeace was my best man and Syd Smith, my good friend from the First Artillery Survey Company and now a returned ex-German POW, a groomsman. Also in attendance were John Wright, my former commanding officer, John Shaw, Jim Armstrong and several members of the 2/15th Field Regiment, as well as other mates who had been POWs. Des, Syd and I were all in uniform. The next day Beth and I packed our bags into the boot of Donald and drove north towards Tea Gardens for our honeymoon.

One lasting memory I have of our wedding is the sound of bagpipes. Beth, being of Scottish descent, decided we should have a piper for the occasion. I remember there was a cemetery right next to the church and before the ceremony he was walking up and down, practising — stirring up the ghosts with his pipes. It proved to be a good omen: we have now been married for 58 years.

AFTER RETURNING HOME FROM captivity, I endeavoured to expand Part 2 of my original diary (the one returned to me by John Shaw). I spent many nights trying to reconstruct my past with help from a friend I had known since the 1930s, Mary Best, who could type at talking speed. My expanded diary covered the period from Christmas Day 1942 to January 1944. What I wrote wasn't personal: just the facts, all of which I committed to paper with a sense of cool detachment.

The medical records Jim Armstrong returned were of help, but there was still so much missing from before 1942. It wasn't until my buried diary summary was returned to me — tucked inside that large brown envelope from the War Graves Services — on 15 February 1947, the fifth anniversary of the fall of Singapore — that I felt I had enough material to keep going with my writing. It would one day form the essential basis of this memoir.

In the meantime, I was very busy with life and realising my ambitions. In 1947, the year of my marriage to Beth, I was working as a Junior Resident Medical Officer at the Crown Street Women's Hospital, Sydney, as well as studying obstetrics and gynaecology. I then spent a year as a research fellow with the National Health and Medical Research Council at Crown Street. In 1949 our first son, David, was born, shortly after I had commenced private practice in Seaforth, just as I had aspired to do when I had been in captivity. With the assistance of John Shaw, who lived in the adjacent suburb of Balgowlah, I set about designing a house based on the plans John had helped me draw in Burma. It was considerably more modest than our original design — it certainly didn't feature a medical wing! — but it was, nonetheless, the dream home I had always hoped for. The house was built in Balgowlah Heights, overlooking Sydney's Middle Harbour. I spotted the block when returning from a house call to a patient and still clearly recall paying a two-pound deposit at a time when Beth and I were financially strapped. We named the house Duart in honour of Beth's Scottish heritage[6] (the chief of her clan lives at Duart Castle on the Isle of Mull). My dream house served as our family home for more than 43 years.

Our second son, Ian, arrived in 1953. Life was good; very good. It sometimes amazed me how rapidly I overcame my fears of being able to resume a civilised life, but I can now see how I did this. Just as in captivity, I buried myself in work — at the hospital, with my family at home, and I was also engaged in ongoing military service with the Citizen's Military Force (CMF) — first in the Reserve of Officers and then with an artillery unit. I was too busy moving forwards to allow my mind the freedom to roam into darker territory from my past, and I think this was perhaps true for a number of returned soldiers.

For many former prisoners of war, their determination to survive became, on our return home, a determination to succeed: in our families, at work and in the community. It took great courage for men to cope with small children who had not known a father, with wives who had difficulty accepting a changed husband, and into a community that had been indoctrinated with the belief that we had been mutilated physically and mentally by our captors. It also took courage for those with irreparable physical and mental trauma to adjust to their disabilities and society. For the majority, however, it became a challenge: compensating for the 'lost years' by study, hard work and dogged resolve. As a result of their experience in facing and overcoming problems as POWs, most were well equipped to deal with the problems of postwar rehabilitation. Most did not seek sympathy, in fact they rejected it; they relied on themselves and their mates and families for support, and just got on with living — to great effect. (Witness the large numbers of former POWs who became knights, judges and leaders in business, politics and community life.) Counselling and what we now recognise as post-traumatic stress were, at the time, unknown, although deferred pay, rehabilitation and retraining courses, provision of tools of trade, ex-service housing and disability pensions all definitely helped.

The efforts of many well-meaning advocates for special recognition and compensation for 'disabled' ex-prisoners of war were often counterproductive. Some businesses were hesitant to employ ex-prisoners of war because of tags such as 'disabled'. Many men I knew wanted to be left to prove that they were as good as, or better than, their contemporaries, despite their undeniable disabilities. Their success was evidence of their courage and commitment to succeed. There was comfort in the knowledge that the toughness we had developed in captivity would help us cope with any bad patch in our lives as civilians. What steel was in the character of all men had certainly been tempered in the forge of POW life.

MY EXPERIENCES IN CAPTIVITY shaped most, if not all, of my postwar activities. Possibly more than anything else, my time as a prisoner of war taught me how to adapt. In civilian life this gave me the ability to dream up concepts, plan and then implement them. I returned from the war with the knowledge, confidence and passion to search for new answers to problems, as well as a lifelong commitment to preventive health and medicine. And, just as surgeon Bertie Coates had told me when I saw him at the 55 Kilo camp all those years ago, I realised that I had truly developed the ability to intuitively know when a patient needed help.

During my time in the CMF — between 1946 and 1971 — I had a number of commanding officers come to see me under the guise of a trivial medical problem (I recall one patient visiting me with a pimple on his nose). I recognised these men were feeling poorly not for physical reasons but because they were lonely. As commanding officers they had no one to talk to: they couldn't talk to their majors because they were breathing down their necks for a promotion, and they certainly couldn't show any signs of weakness to their men, so I found myself in a role of confidant. What they needed was private guidance, something I gradually came to understand I had already been giving for years.

My extraordinary past always seemed to influence how I approached any new challenge in my life back home. While I do not want this final chapter to turn into a curriculum vitae, I will detail, with brevity, my career path after the war in an attempt to convey just how greatly one's past can mould a future.

In 1960, I joined the St John Ambulance Association, where I was deeply involved in standardising first-aid training programs for the organisation's examinations and ultimately designed the St John First-Aid Kits based on the Army first-aid kits we had issued to our own men before going into action in Malaya. My own experience in action had helped me to realise just how few items were actually essential. In the mid-1960s I became very interested in sports training and medicine via my elder son, David, who had a passion for rowing throughout high school. Searching for answers to problems David's rowing team was experiencing, I developed a new style of fitness program concentrating on both aerobic and strength training, and then progressed to designing a different style of rowing focused on far greater strength in the arms relative to strength in the legs. In short, this same program was adopted by the Sydney Rowing Club eight which won the Kings Cup and were then selected as the 1968 Olympic eight.

My interest in schoolboy rowing became more serious when I was subsequently selected as medical advisor for the Australian Olympic rowing teams for the Mexico Games in 1968 and Munich in 1972. (There is, of course, another story here about Munich, with the dreadful fate of the Israeli Olympic team members murdered by terrorists during the Games, but that is not my story to tell. I was merely one of thousands there watching at the time.)

Mentally, my war and captivity experiences always seemed to be helping or influencing me, but physical problems from my past eventually became more than a hindrance, forcing my medical career to take a new turn in 1966. By the 1960s I was suffering worsening psoriasis. This skin condition started developing mildly in captivity, probably due to malnutrition and stress, but became increasingly worse over the years. One of the complications of psoriasis is psoriatic arthritis, which caused me to lose dexterity and also became a significant hygiene issue. Before operating I had to scrub thoroughly, and my hands eventually reached the point where every time I scrubbed they would bleed.

With no choice but to retire from surgery, I searched for alternative challenges and became very excited about what was then a new field of medical care: executive health. Again, prevention was the key. Most senior executives in the postwar period were ex-servicemen and they'd quickly become used to living hard and playing hard. After returning home from years of deprivation, a lot of these men had been behaving like kids in a lolly shop. Many were cutting the unhealthy figure of a bald, overweight smoker. They were extremely intelligent when it came to their careers, but when it came to their health, they needed a lot of persuasion. Initially employed by Ampol as a consultant, my job was to educate these men about becoming self-reliant with their health. At each consultation I found myself having to almost con executives into eating more wisely, stopping smoking, starting exercise programs, reducing their cholesterol and learning to control stress (a scenario which doctors today still have to play out with their patients). This new role, part-time in conjunction with my practice, took me to London, Toronto and San Francisco to visit clinics to study other executive health programs. Eventually, I rented a private room in the Ampol building in North Sydney, with Beth as my assistant,[7] and by 1972 I was practising executive health full-time, which I continued to do until I retired in 2000.

While I missed surgery, I found great pleasure in the varied directions my life took as a result. At the same time as I pursued executive health I also remained committed to sports medicine, becoming president of the NSW branch of the Australian Sports Medicine Foundation between 1976 and 1978, and medical director of the Sydney City to Surf Fun Run between 1977 and 1998. During this time I researched the cause and control of heat exhaustion, again, and as always, assisted by Beth. In 1998, at 82 years of age, I stepped down as honorary medical director after 21 years, becoming honorary medical consultant. My son David, a cardiologist and the deputy medical director of the race, was appointed as my replacement. The City to Surf role became, and remains, one of my greatest passions: it involves everything I love most in life — my family, medicine, research and the celebration and promotion of health and fitness.

WHILE IT IS HAS only been in recent years that I have allowed previously controlled emotions to surface, this process of unravelling, albeit slowly, was unquestionably helped by a series of journeys, four of which were especially significant.

By early 1946, when the British Commonwealth Occupation Force (BCOF) was in Japan, I had begun writing to both Matsumoto and Takahashi. One of Beth's nursing friends, Joan Mills (Beth's chief bridesmaid), was a member of the BCOF, and I sent money to her with a request to regularly buy food parcels for my two friends in Sakata, whom I knew would be doing it tough in the aftermath of Japan's defeat. It was my turn to repay their kindness. I received letters from both, thanking me for the food parcels and we maintained in regular contact, hoping that one day we would have the opportunity to see each other again. In 1959, that opportunity arose when I was appointed as RMO to a Landing Ship Medium (LSM) being brought back from Japan for the Army, and I booked a ticket for Beth to join me there.

Perhaps strangely to some, I did not feel any hesitation about returning to Japan. Years had passed and all that was on my mind was the chance to see my friends again. I remember our train pulling into Sakata and spotting Matsumoto and Takahashi waiting on the platform, flanked by their wives and children. My two friends looked much the same as I remembered them, although, naturally, a little older. They greeted us with Oriental reserve, as effusive as they could be. I met them with a huge smile and equally polite greetings in my best phrase-book Japanese — having quickly forgotten so much of the language I had learned during captivity.

Our stay proved to be a moving reunion which gave me the chance to visit familiar places, including the billets where we had spent such a miserable winter, the crematorium to which many of the bodies of our men had been sent, and Honmer's Garden, the charming Japanese sanctuary Mrs Narita had taken me to following the end of the war. We talked little of the past and mostly of our families and my men. They were keen to hear news of Kitch Loughnan and Butch Hall, two of Takahashi's assistants at the butchery during our time in Sakata. I was able to report that Kitch had returned to a career in grazing back in Queensland, and Butch was running his own business as a butcher in Sydney.

Throughout our visit, I was cheerful on the surface — genuinely pleased to see my friends again, as they were to see me — but inside I was aware of a struggle to calm stirred emotions. As always, I won the battle, carefully managing to keep my feelings at bay by focusing on the purpose of my trip: the chance to personally thank these men for their help so long ago. At the beginning of our visit, I had tried to return the beautiful kimono Takahashi had given me for 'happy occasions' before we parted ways in Sakata, but he refused to accept it. However, both men were willing to accept the plush koalas Beth and I had brought over from Australia for them. When I presented my friends with the koalas I said: 'Thank you for your kindness to me and my men, at great personal risk. I have never forgotten you.'

The fact that their compassion had been such a rarity at the time had made their acts all the greater, and I assured my friends I would always remember them. For me this visit represented a debt fulfilled.

Further journeys were not made until much later in my life. In 1992, when I was 76 years old, I joined a pilgrimage to Singapore and was invited to give an address at the 50th Anniversary of the fall of Singapore Commemoration. Again accompanied by Beth, I visited Gemas, Muar, Tamarkan and Kanchanaburi. I viewed the visit as a chance for a catharsis of sorts, but went to great pains to ensure my address did not tap into areas that might send me into uncharted emotions. Six years later, I joined a Department of Veterans' Affairs pilgrimage to the opening of the Hellfire Pass Memorial Museum by Prime Minister John Howard. Again, feelings about my past stirred and I suppressed them — until Anzac Day. When the 'Last Post' was sounded at the first light of dawn, the Hellfire Pass illuminated only by candles, there was not a dry eye amongst us. The sound of the 'Last Post' always brings me undone.

Having Beth with me undoubtedly made the first two of these journeys (and others I will not go into here[8]) far easier. I am an extremely private person but nobody knows me better than Beth, not even my former prisoner-of-war mates. Over our years together I have been able to talk to her about my past — not in any great detail, and, until recently, always without emotion — but the fact that we could at least talk prevented a barrier between us from ever being present (something I am aware has ruined the marriages of other former prisoners of war). Whenever I spoke to Beth about my days in captivity, I think she knew there was always more to a particular story than what I'd stated, and she seemed to understand. In reality, Beth probably learned more about my past from my friends, such as Des Makepeace and John Shaw, than she did from me, but the important thing was that she never pushed me. That understanding between us became even greater as the years of our marriage passed, and I will always be grateful to her for this. Our trips to Sakata, Singapore, Malaysia and Thailand gave Beth the opportunity to see for herself the setting of many of the stories she had heard from my friends and I had relayed to her, and with each journey I was able to reveal to her a little more about my history.

My final significant journey into my past took place in 2003 when I returned to Thailand and Burma. Unfortunately Beth was not able to accompany me: after undergoing four spinal fusion operations, three operations for a fractured hip and replacement of both shoulders, overseas travel was no longer an option for her. This time my travel companions were our sons, David, then aged 53, and Ian, aged 49.

In Thailand we visited Bangkok, Kanburi, the Hellfire Pass and the Three Pagodas Pass, and in Burma we visited Rangoon and, most importantly for me, Thanbyuzayat — where my Railway journey had begun, and Hlepauk (18 Kilo camp). Burma was where I really wanted to go because that was where most of my men had been buried. At 86 years of age, I knew this trip would be my last bite at the cherry, so to speak. I wanted to pay my final respects to my fallen comrades.

My sons already knew plenty about my past — they had read the various versions of my expanded diaries — but their knowledge had limited meaning until we made this trip together. We were part of a tour group led by Lieutenant Colonel Terry Beaton (Retired); including me there were four veterans in our travelling group of about 90, and the younger members of the group constantly and sensitively quizzed us about our past experiences at each location. Being on the ground in Thailand and Burma, retracing some of my steps, informed my sons more than either had ever garnered from books. Now they could see for themselves where I had been and understand just how black nights in the tropics can be, how hot and how humid. Again, it seemed very little needed to be said between us, they could feel the heat, so to speak, and, like Beth, they seemed to understand.

Upon our return home, Beth and I were both surprised that neither David nor Ian spoke much about the trip: I think they were stunned, but it definitely brought us closer together in a tacit way. At the 2/15th Field Regiment reunion following our trip, I asked David to be our MC for the evening and after the formalities were over I noticed that he became very choked up — as was Ian when he proposed a toast to the veterans. I think that was when I realised how much our sons had learned and been affected by our journey together. Each of us returned home with the capacity to acknowledge my past experiences in a new and intimate way.

I DO NOT CLAIM that my own experiences postwar represent how all returned former POWs coped with civilian life. For some, their period in action and captivity remained a nightmare they experienced over and over again, a manifestation of post-traumatic stress disorder; while for others, the lid was closed, horrible memories forced to fade into the background and their lives were somehow moved on, kept forever busy.

I have always lived my life in compartments, and perhaps this helped me to get on with the job of living, both during and after captivity. All my life I have only ever been capable of opening one box at a time, dealing with a particular situation or event, and then closing it — sometimes permanently — before moving on to whatever is waiting for me in the next little box in line. I try not to agonise over choices: I prefer to make a decision and then rule a line in the ledger so I can move forward with a clear mind. I have consciously chosen to live a life without continually glancing backwards.

In writing this memoir, my editor has constantly been asking me how I *felt* about certain situations, events and memories from my past. It ultimately became a point of humour between us, as she tried to reword her questions to avoid using the word 'feel'; trying desperately to make me drop my guard — but there was no guard in place. In most cases I couldn't recall my feelings because I simply hadn't experienced them. Of course, as I have already written, my upbringing made me a reserved and somewhat introverted man, but during my years in captivity I can now see I became almost blindingly objective. What took place in those years under the merciless rule of the IJA was a process of desensitisation. Until recently, I have thought little of it. I did not realise my lack of emotion might be seen as curious or even unbelievable by others who had not lived through experiences similar to mine.

POW life severely damaged, even destroyed, almost all of my sensitivities. It has taken time — more than 50 years — for them to come close to being repaired. (And I am referring to emotional responses in general, not only memories of my time in captivity: it has only been in recent years that I have been able to shed tears when reading a poignant book, watching a film or learning of the passing of a loved one.)

The writing of my story has certainly helped, as too has the passing of time. Perhaps losing so many of my mates in later years of my life, especially Des Makepeace and John Shaw, has also softened my reserve. Without as many mates to share that unspoken understanding maybe I have gradually been able to dig deeper, my defences pierced so I can again revisit some of the more painful shards of my past, but again I cannot say for sure.

I am still at times bewildered that others have expressed interest in my experiences of captivity — after all, in strictly factual terms, they constitute only three and a half years of my 89 years of life. But now, at the very end of writing this book, when I look back and consider how these years have affected the rest of my life, perhaps it is not so strange after all.

EPILOGUE

I have written my story because I believe the memory of veterans forms a vast repository of knowledge and experience which should be passed on to the present and future generations, with the hope of providing a better understanding of where our nation has come from and perhaps even in which directions it is heading. My challenge has been to communicate my own memories as clearly, accurately and emotionally honestly as I am capable. Writing this book has honoured a sense of duty towards my comrades, and it represents a desire fulfilled.

I can honestly say that had I known what was in store for me on the day I set sail out of Sydney Harbour back in 1941, I never would have had the guts to face up to it. Having survived, I wouldn't have missed any of it for the world. Throughout my time in action and captivity I was able to inject very real meaning into my life — and those experiences made all of my postwar achievements, happiness and dreams possible.

THE STORY OF JOHN BULL:
AN IMPORTANT TRIBUTE

During the final days of the Malayan campaign in February 1942, many of us maintained hope that, maybe, just maybe, there would be a rescue attempt, but this was nothing more than wishful thinking. A small group of us led by our 2 i/c John Workman, with the assistance of Ted Dahl, the 84 LAD engineer, and Stuart Ward, the adjutant — and with the blessing of our CO Lieutenant Colonel John Wright — made plans to prepare boats in the event of an evacuation Dunkirk-style, to enable the 2/15th to remain intact as a unit.

On 12 February, orders were issued by one of the battery commanders to two of his battery officers to seek, obtain and prepare sufficient transport to provide for the whole regiment in the event of an organised evacuation. Two of the officers, Lieutenant John Bull and Lieutenant Roger Martin, along with some of their sergeants and other men, found two suitable small island cargo ships about 30 metres long, which they believed would be adequate for the task. They were coal burner steamers with a bridge, a small cargo hold fore and aft and the decks covered by canvas awnings. One of the boats, the *Hong Tat*, under the control of John Bull, was soon made ready, and with a little work the engines were made efficient and effective. The engines on the other ship, however, could not be repaired, and Roger Martin returned to Regimental Headquarters to obtain assistance from the engineers to repair his ship. During action, the last we heard was that John Bull and his troops on the *Hong Tat* had been raked by machine-gun fire while they were moored just off the end of the pier — but there would be a lot more to learn about this event in years to come.

At a regimental meeting in the early 1980s, called to discuss this event, John Bull told us the complete story of what happened. Following the machine-gun fire, which killed one of our men, Bull weighed anchor and pulled further out into Keppel Harbour. He then came back to the pier area and found a naval commander, the RN chief naval officer in charge of evacuation. By this time the chaotic evacuation of Singapore was well under way for civilians and certain selected military personnel. Bull was told that the Japanese were just around the corner and held most of the eastern area of the docks. The RN commander ordered him to take what men he could — in addition to his original group — and wished him the best of luck. John Bull, realising he would be unable to make further contact with the 2/15th, followed these orders. He and his party, now increased to 26 men, were heading for minefields when they were warned by a small RN patrol boat that they were in potential danger. The naval patrol issued Bull with a chart and guided him out of the harbour.

After some days and many harrowing experiences, including being bombed, they reached Sumatra, travelled at night, and then arrived at the Sunda Straits about the time that a Japanese fleet destroyed HMAS *Perth*, the USS *Houston*, and other Allied vessels in the battle of the Sunda Straits. A small Japanese naval frigate stopped Bull and he was ordered to follow the frigate to the tiny Banka Island (near Sumatra). Bull and his party endured some three months here as prisoners before being taken to Palembang, in Sumatra, where they spent the rest of the war in Japanese captivity.

After the war was over, Bull went to the Palembang aerodrome and, with a few of his troops, took the surrender of the Japanese officers and 300 men and notified Mountbatten's headquarters in Singapore. Within hours, Lady Mountbatten had arrived to inspect the POWs.

Bull and his party were then taken to Changi where they were ostracised by the officers and men of their own regiment who believed they had 'deserted'. Nobody asked them what had happened or why they had left before capitulation. Bull and his men were so bitterly disappointed they offered no information. Neither Bull nor his sergeant nor some of the men who were with him have ever attended a regimental reunion.

At no stage were John Bull and his original group of men deserters. They behaved with the highest standard of discipline, comradeship and integrity. Bull lost only three men from his group in three and a half years. This can only be explained by his resourcefulness and efficiency in maintaining morale and cohesion. Bull's sergeant was Jim Fitzhardinge and the engineer who repaired the engines, and subsequently drove them, was Charlie Ericsson. This tale is a sad commentary on a lack of communication and understanding; reference is made here to exonerate Bull and his men who were never deserters. They were, in fact, deserted by some of their own officers and men.

ENDNOTES

Chapter Two — Australia at war

1   This new brigade joined the 22nd and 23rd Brigades to form the 8th Division (one of four divisions of the Second AIF to serve in the Second World War). The 2/15th Field Regiment was the last AIF field regiment to be formed in the Second World War.

Chapter Three — Bound for action

1   Moremon, Dr John, with Reid, Dr Richard, 2002, pp. 2–3.
2   For readers not familiar with 'military establishment', our regiment, at this point in time, was made up of Regimental Headquarters and two batteries, with each battery incorporating three troops. The 29th Battery consisted of A Troop, B Troop and C Troop, while our 30th Battery consisted of D Troop, E Troop and F Troop. As RMO, I belonged to Regimental Headquarters.
3   Statistics calculated from Cochrane, Peter, 2001, p. 116.
4   'Now is the Hour', lyrics and music by Maewa Kaihan, Clement Scott, Dorothy Stewart, 1913.

Chapter Four — The Malayan campaign

1   The first part of my diary would later be confiscated by the Japanese, but I did manage to retain a summary of this first part. The events of this chapter are based on my summary, and have been verified courtesy 'The Operational Story of 2/15th Field Regiment, 8 Div AIF in the Malayan Campaign, December 5, 1941 to February 18, 1942' by Lieutenant Colonel J.W. Wright, DFC, EM, as published in Whitelocke, Cliff, 1983.
2   Charlton, Peter, 1994, p. 46.

3   The guns were 'under command' of the infantry — located among the forward infantry instead of 'in support', where they would have been positioned well behind the forward troops. In subsequent action the artillery would always remain in support.
4   The 2/19th Battalion and a troop of gunners from the 13th Battery of the 4th Anti-Tank Regiment.
5   The 2/29th Battalion and 2/19th Battalion.
6   I understood that the 2/29th Battalion lost 417 men and that the 2/19th Battalion lost 220 men.
7   Wigmore, Lionel, 1957, p. 247.

Chapter Five — Into captivity

1   It was later reported that Wally Brown and his followers did escape from Singapore. Wally apparently reached Sumatra, Indonesia, where he was separated from his group — who managed to return to Australia — and was not heard of again.
2   Moremon, Dr John, 2003, pp. 8, 142.
3   This list was revised in August 1944 and 66 of the 99 missing were accounted for, including 30 in Java/Sumatra, eight in Australia and 22 in Changi. The nominal roll can be viewed at the AWM in Canberra, reference: PR01966, 2/15th Field Regiment RAA AIF Association.
4   After the war, the 2/15th Field Regiment Association began publishing a newsletter, *Hibiscus Leaves*, originally written with the objective of reporting births. It is still published under this title and is edited by my wife, Beth Richards.
5   Wigmore, Lionel, 1957, p. 519.
6   Bennett successfully escaped home to Australia, where he was given a very cool reception. Bennett claimed he escaped to tell the true story of the Malayan campaign, and to warn Australia of a Japanese attack. In Australia, a Commission of Inquiry found Bennett had wrongfully abandoned his own men. His escape remains a contentious issue in the history of the fallout from the Malayan campaign.
7   Initially Colonel Anderson was senior staff officer to Brigadier Varley but he later replaced Major Don Kerr as commanding officer of No. 2 Battalion, with Don Kerr becoming 2 i/c to Anderson.

Chapter Six — 'A' Force

1   As soon as it was apparent 'A' Force was to be split up, Varley had quickly recognised the need to spread medical resources amongst all the men, so had bolstered the number of medical resources in both Green and Ramsay Forces — his foresight in this regard was rewarded in days to come.

2 Whitecross, Roy H., 1953, p. 35.
3 Prior to captivity, we knew and referred to Thailand as Siam, the country's official name until 1949. However, the Japanese referred to the country as Thailand; hence, we were members of the No. 3 Thai POW camp. Throughout this book, I vary usage between Thailand and Siam, just as we did during captivity — and as recorded in my diary.
4 Excerpts of Nagatomo's speech quoted from Hall, L, 1985, pp. 15–18.

Chapter Seven — Railway life
1 Wigmore, Lionel, 1957, p. 547.
2 This microscope is now held by the AWM, Canberra.
3 The camp canteen operated by buying goods from Burmese traders for reselling to our own men. The profits were used to buy extra rations for the sick, or for special occasions such as this.

Chapter Eight — A new year
1 It should be noted that pellagra has a cyclical history, and it is possible that the improvement in the men was part of the cycle of the disease, but at the time we were all encouraged by the fact that our improvised efforts seemed to be working.
2 A band, with instruments recently arrived from Singapore, from Brigade ('A' Force) Headquarters.

Chapter Nine — Line laying
1 Even the Japanese and Korean guards referred to me as the 'boy' or 'baby' doctor owing to my youthful appearance.

Chapter Ten — A new killer
1 Remarkably, no infections resulted from his poor hygiene.
2 My recollection of this incident has been verified by Hall, L., 1985 (pp. 164–5) and the personal diary of Colonel John Williams (entries for Saturday, 1 May, and Sunday, 2 May 1943).
3 Six hundred men of Anderson Force and 867 of Williams Force, as recorded in the personal diary of Colonel John Williams (entry for Saturday, 8 May 1943).
4 My recollection of this incident has been verified by the personal diary of Colonel John Williams (entry for Saturday, 8 May, 1943).
5 The main isolation staff consisted of Jim Armstrong, Pinkey Rhodes, Bob Kemp, Woodbridge, Arthur Baker, Jack McKone, Harry Moxham, Keith Fisher and Duncan McNaughton of Anderson Force, and Johnson, Kelly

and Kirby of Williams Force. They were assisted in the main camp by Arthur Harris, Don Booth, Don Bertram, Allan Taylor, Jamieson and Waters of Anderson Force and Miles of Williams Force. (Note: I did not record the names of all orderlies in my diary, and some only by surname.)

6   When the last of the smallpox cases at the 45 Kilo camp had been cleared, the patients had been returned to Fitzsimmons Force, while Dr Hekking and Bill Drower had been sent back to headquarters at Thanbyuzayat.

7   Five of these deaths were from Anderson Force, as recorded in Anderson Force medical records kept by Jim Armstrong, and also recorded in my diary, Papers of Dr Rowley Richards, AWM PR01916, Canberra. The other three were from Williams Force, as recorded in my diary only. There may have been more from Williams Force, but I do not have the official records of Williams Force to verify this figure.

8   I have realised, postwar, that this philosophy was encapsulated in an Alcoholics' Anonymous Prayer, which I remember as 'God, grant me the serenity to accept the things I cannot change, the courage to change the things I can, and the wisdom to know the difference.'

9   As recorded in my original diary, 9 June (Taunzan), Papers of Dr Rowley Richards, AWM PR01916, Canberra.

10 As recorded in my original diary, 13 July (Taunzan), Papers of Dr Rowley Richards, AWM PR01916, Canberra.

11 As recorded in my original diary, 13 July (Taunzan), Papers of Dr Rowley Richards, AWM PR01916, Canberra.

Chapter Eleven — Death camps
1   Whitecross, Roy H., 1953, p. 86.
2   Blair, Clay, Interview.
3   As recorded in Anderson Force medical records kept by Jim Armstrong, Papers of Dr Rowley Richards, AWM PR01916, Canberra.
4   Diary entry for Thursday, 9 September, 1943, Papers of Dr Rowley Richards, AWM PR01916, Canberra.

Chapter Twelve — A brief respite
1   Some history books record the date of the Railway being joined as 16 October, others 17 October. In my diary I recorded the date as 17 October.
2   Moremon, Dr John, 2003, p. 86.

Chapter Thirteen — New journeys
1   Our battalion initially consisted of approximately 1000 men, but 250 were sent from Tavoy to Ye and some others left Anderson Force in

southern Burma due to sickness. Hence, my records show the total strength of Anderson Force at the beginning of the Railway as 739 men.

2   Hall, L., 1985, p. 271: quoted from 'Letter of Condolence on the Occasion of the Memorial Service for Deceased POWs', 20 November, 1943.

3   The spelling of place names was often inconsistent owing to English translations. We also knew Non Pladuk as Nong Pladuk and Nonproduck.

4   I have no recollection of Christmas in this 'land of plenty'; nor did I make any mention of Christmas celebrations in my diary at the time. I cannot explain why.

Chapter Fourteen — Buried treasure

1   From an old Russian proverb, 'unless you have supped from the same bowl, you cannot know the taste'.

2   Years after the war, Peter sent me a personal note of thanks and a cheque for $1000 for the 2/15th Field Regiment Association funds. His note read: 'To repay a debt incurred in a [rail] truck in Malaya.'

Chapter Fifteen — All at sea

1   Along with other men who survived the *Rakuyo Maru*, I remember this tanker being hit. However, in my travels to Washington postwar to examine official documents in the Naval Archives, there is no record to support this version of events. An error in the records, or our memories playing tricks again? I cannot say for certain.

Chapter Sixteen — Rescued

1   Savage, Russell, 1995, p. 83.

2   Blair, Joan and Clay, 1979, p. 291; Savage, Russell, 1995, p. 87.

3   Barrett, Peirce, Pote-Hunt, Richards, Roulston, 'Report on Prisoners of War Camp: Sakata', 30 August 1945. Copy available within Papers of Dr Rowley Richards, AWM PR01916, Australian War Memorial, Canberra.

4   *Ibid.*

5   It was not until the 1970s, when I was interviewed by authors Clay and Joan Blair for their book *Return from the River Kwai* that I was told this mother whaling ship was actually loaded with crude oil. We were sitting on dynamite the whole time. Ignorance was most certainly bliss and I remain grateful we were not aware of this during our journey.

6   Wigmore, Lionel, 1957, p. 615.

Chapter Seventeen — Sakata

1   Some of the material from this chapter has been drawn from a report on Sakata I wrote with Captain Barrett and Captain Roulston entitled: 'Report on Prisoners of War Camp: Sakata', 30th August 1945. The report was signed by: Captain J.E. ('Tam') Peirce (RA); Captain R. Pote-Hunt (RA); Captain C.W. Barrett (Int. Corps); Captain J.R. Roulston (RAMC) and me (AAMC).

2   'See you Toosday' was a family saying. I included reference to this in any messages home to establish authenticity.

Chapter Eighteen — Liberation at last

1   I recorded what I could remember of his speech in my notebook later that day, as per this quote.

2   Quoted directly from a copy of the original note, as recorded in my notebook.

3   At the time, 'legation' was the term used to signify a diplomatic representative office of less importance than an embassy. Following the Second World War, the distinction between an embassy and a legation was abandoned.

Epilogue

1   In Manila we rested in an American convalescent hospital, where we met some Australian nurses, one of whom was Veronica Tapprell whom I had known at Ingleburn camp before we left Australia. Our interaction with these nurses was a critical transition point: we had long been fearing we might never again adjust to civilised society, but within hours we were rapidly resuming life — talking comfortably with the nurses and obtaining supplies of beer, gin and whisky, which were on issue as part of the convalescent 'diet', together with a weekly carton of cigarettes, a Yellow Bowl pipe (one of the best brands) and pipe tobacco, plus the mandatory ice-cream. We were having parties just as we had done in Sydney years ago, carrying on where we had left off.

2   Each of these men was genuine in his belief that I had died. It is another example of contaminated memory.

3   During my stopover in Manila I had sent a special cheerio wireless message to the nuns at the Mater at a time of night when they should have been tucked up in their cots. The nuns had apparently heard my message and had always been very interested in my whereabouts during the war. My visit to the nuns was important to me because I wanted to

repay their kindness and concern. When I arrived they greeted me with a very special 'welcome home' feast — it was a great occasion, especially as I was not one of 'their mob'.

4   These letters were written during late 1942 and 1943 as 'letters home' to describe in detail my experiences.

5   While neither Beth nor I were religious we both lived by Christian ethics and alternatives to church weddings were not considered at the time.

6   To this day I still affectionately refer to Beth as my pig-headed Scot!

7   While Beth accompanied me, as 'Rowley's wife', in my activities, I also accompanied her, as 'Beth's husband', in her activities as Regional President and member of the International Toastmistress Clubs.

8   In the late 1970s, accompanied by Beth, I visited Singapore, Malaysia and Thailand to retrace my steps in especially significant places such as Gemas, Muar, Parit Sulong, Tanglin, Changi, Tamarkan and Kanchanaburi. In 1981 I visited Washington, DC, to study records, particularly relating to the shipwreck and the recovery of survivors, in the National Archives of the US and the US Navy Archives. Some of the photos taken on the trips were published in my first book, *The Survival Factor* (1989).

BIBLIOGRAPHY

Blair, Joan and Blair, Clay, 1978, Interviews with Rowley Richards for research for *Return From the River Kwai* (1979).

——1979, *Return From the River Kwai*, Raven (Macdonald General Books), London

Canfield, Michael and Nolan, Patrick, 2002, Interviews with Rowley Richards for 'Australians At War' Archives, Department of Veterans' Affairs, Canberra

Charlton, Peter, 1994, 'The Retreat from Malaya', pages 46–52 in Horner, Dr David, 1994, *The Battles that Shaped Australia* (*The Australian* series), Allen & Unwin, Sydney

Cochrane, Peter, 2001, *Australians at War*, ABC Books, Sydney

Day, David, 2003, *The Politics of War*, HarperCollins*Publishers*, Sydney

Denton, Andrew, 2004, 'ANZAC Day Special' *Enough Rope*, (transcript of interview with Rowley Richards), ABC Television

Department of Veterans' Affairs, 2002, *Stolen Years: Australian Prisoners of War*, Commonwealth Department of Communications, Canberra

Hall, Leslie, 1985, *The Blue Haze: Incorporating a History of 'A' Force — Groups 3–5*, Sutton & Co., Australia

Horner, Dr David, 1994, *The Battles that Shaped Australia* (*The Australian* series), Allen & Unwin, Sydney

Loughnan, Kitchener ('Kitch'), M., extracts from the personal diary of Kitchener Loughnan, loaned to me by his sons Harry and Bill (unpublished)

Lynch, James ('Jim'), P., extracts from the personal diary of James P. Lynch, loaned to me by his sister Mrs Kath Harrison (unpublished)

Maher, Francis, S. ('Scippy'), extracts from the personal diary of Francis S. Maher, loaned to me by his widow, Mrs Joan Maher (unpublished)

BIBLIOGRAPHY

Moremon, Dr John, 2003, *Australians on the Burma–Thailand Railway 1942–43*, Department of Veterans' Affairs, Canberra.

Moremon, Dr John, with Reid, Dr Richard, 2002, *A Bitter Fate: Australians in Malaya & Singapore*, December 1941–February 1942, Department of Veterans' Affairs, Canberra

Orman, Alison, May 2004–March 2005, Interviews with Dr Rowley Richards, Mrs Beth Richards and F.J. ('Pinkey') Rhodes (unpublished)

Richards, Rowley, 'Papers of Dr Rowley Richards' (including parts of original wartime diaries and buried diary summary and medical records, known as the Rowley Richards Collection, AWM PR01916), Canberra

——1999, 'The Importance of Veteran Memory', public address delivered on 28 October 1999, Department of Veterans' Affairs Conference, Powerhouse Museum, Sydney

Richards, Rowley and McEwan, Marcia, 1989, *The Survival Factor*, Kangaroo Press, Kenthurst, Sydney

Savage, Russell, 1995, *A Guest of the Emperor*, Boolarong Press, Moorooka, Queensland

2/15th Field Regiment RAA AIF Association, Papers of 2/15 Field Regiment RAA AIF Association, AWM PR01966, Canberra.

Shaw, John, extracts from the personal diary of Major J.A.L. Shaw, DSO, loaned to me by Mary Shaw, wife of John Shaw's late son, David (unpublished)

Whitecross, Roy H., extracts from the personal diaries of Roy Whitecross, loaned to me by the author (unpublished)

——1953, *Slaves of the Son of Heaven: The Personal Story of an Australian Prisoner of the Japanese During the Years 1942–1945*, Dymocks Book Arcade, Sydney

Whitelocke, Cliff, 1983, *Gunners in the Jungle: A Story of the 2/15th Field Regiment Royal Australian Artillery, 8th Division, Australian Imperial Force*, 2/15th Field Regiment Association, Sydney

Williams, John, extracts from the personal diary of Lieutenant Colonel John Williams, OBE, ED (unpublished)

Wigmore, Lionel, 1957, *Australia in the War of 1939–1945: The Japanese Thrust*, Australian War Memorial, Canberra

INDEX

Bashford, Padre, 92,
182–183
bashings
within Japanese Army,
109, 126, 131–132,
135–136, 210
at Little Nike,
192–193
of Mills, 146
Naito orders, 139, 141
by Nippon Tsun
Company, 251, 252
of officers, 91
of RR, 109–110,
213–214
on Singapore docks,
83
of Williams, 124, 148,
185, 215
Beaton, Lieutenant
Colonel Terry, 302
Bennett, Lieutenant
General Gordon
commands 8th
Division AIF, 57
escapes from
Singapore, 67, 80,
95, 310
issues orders to
surrender, 67, 69
beriberi
at Hlepauk, 106
at Little Nike, 195
at Sakata, 250,
256–257
at Selarang Barracks,
78
at Tan Yin, 119
at Taunzan, 158
Best, Mary, 294
Bible, 94
Birdwood Camp
(Changi) see under
Changi
Black, Lieutenant
Colonel Chris,
177, 182
Black Force, 177
black market, 78, 96, 110
Blazey, Barbara, 26, 178
board and lodging, 96,
110

body lice, 255–256
Booth, Don, 81, 86–87,
133, 164, 199, 204
brewer's yeast, 108
'Bridge Over the River
Kwai', 196
British Army see also
Royal Navy
2nd Loyals Battalion,
61–62
No. 2 Mobile Force,
175
AIF conforms to, 58
Anglo-American
Force, 133, 145
in Changi Gaol, 72
history, 50
hygiene see under
hygiene
International Red
Cross, 257
on Kachidoki Maru,
221, 241–242
on Kibitsu Maru,
242–243, 246
medical officers, 51
officers' privileges see
under officers'
privileges
POWs, 89, 104, 145,
206, 276
smallpox see under
smallpox
at Tamarkan camp, 197
British Commonwealth
Occupation Force
(BCOF), 299
Britz, Sergeant Peter, 209
Brown, Sergeant Wally,
70, 310
Buchan, John, 180–181
bugle calls, 98, 147–148,
301
Bukit Timah (Singapore),
79
Bull, Lieutenant John,
306–308
Burgess, Lieutenant
Lloyd, 146
Burke, Jim, 230
Burma, 85, 87, 97, 117,
178, 236, 302

native Burmese, 96,
104, 149, 155, 164,
167, 184
Burma–Siam Railway
No. 1 Branch Thai
POW camp, 206
No. 3 Branch Thai
POW camp, 98,
195, 196, 197, 198
No. 5 Branch Thai
POW camp,
168–171, 195, 196,
197, 198
Thanbyuzayat (0 Kilo
camp) see
Thanbyuzayat
(Burma)
14 Kilo camp, 133
Hlepauk (18 Kilo
camp), 102,
103–116, 302
Kunknitkway (26 Kilo
camp), 102,
129–141, 142–143,
144
Retpu (30 Kilo
hospital camp),
102, 127–128, 134,
145, 171, 175,
176–183, 193
Tan Yin (35 Kilo
camp), 102,
116–128
40 Kilo camp, 155, 164
Anarkwan (45 Kilo
camp), 102,
144–148, 164
55 Kilo camp hospital,
102, 162, 163,
164–165, 171, 182,
188, 197, 296
Taunzan (60 Kilo
camp), 102, 144,
147–148, 149–160,
161, 162, 164, 176
62 Kilo camp, 175
68 Kilo peg, 161
Mizale (70 Kilo
camp), 102, 159,
161, 163–167, 171
Apparon (80 Kilo
camp), 102,
167–174, 184